AIDS HEALTH SERVICES AT THE CROSSROADS: LESSONS FOR COMMUNITY CARE

Victoria D. Weisfeld, *Editor*

A Publication of
The Robert Wood Johnson Foundation
Communications Office

Thomas P. Gore II, *Vice President for Communications*
Vivian E. Fransen, *Contributing Editor*
Joan K. Hollendonner, *Production Coordinator*

Princeton, New Jersey

December 1991

Since 1972, The Robert Wood Johnson Foundation, Princeton, New Jersey, has been one of the largest private philanthropies in the United States and is the nation's largest devoted to improving the health and health care of Americans.

Founded as a small local philanthropy in 1936 by General Robert Wood Johnson, the foundation assumed national stature when a major portion of General Johnson's estate was donated to it upon his death in 1968.

With assets of more than $3 billion today, the foundation concentrates its grantmaking in these areas:

to assure that Americans of all ages have access to basic health care;

to improve the way services are organized and provided to people with chronic health conditions;

to promote health and prevent disease by reducing harm caused by substance abuse; and

to help the nation deal with the problem of rising health care costs.

The late General Robert Wood Johnson served from the 1930s to the early 1960s as chairman and chief executive officer of Johnson & Johnson, the health and medical care products company founded by his father and uncle. The foundation, although not a part of Johnson & Johnson, has continued its founder's interest in the health care field.

Library of Congress Catalog Card Number: 91-67786

ISBN 0-942054-04-0

The Robert Wood Johnson Foundation
College Road
Post Office Box 2316
Princeton, NJ 08543-2316
(609) 452-8701

Table of Contents

ACKNOWLEDGEMENTS

A number of individuals deserve thanks for their valuable contributions
to this book. First, those who reviewed the entire manuscript: Debbie
Lamm, Phil Lee, Cliff Morrison, Merv Silverman, Ruby Hearn, and Paul
Jellinek. Pat Franks was especially helpful in interpreting the Ryan
White Comprehensive AIDS Resources Emergency Act legislation. Their
insightful comments and thoughtful suggestions did much to enhance
the text.

Fred Jordan conducted initial interviews for the book and
prepared an early manuscript draft. His role in the first stages of this
project and the enthusiasm he displayed are appreciated.

Special thanks to Andy Burness for the wealth of information
he provided for the media chapter. His practical tips to guide media
relations activities constitute a mini-course for the reader.

Finally, our deep appreciation goes to all of the people
mentioned in the text, whose names and affiliations are listed in the back
of the book. Virtually all of these individuals participated in interviews,
everyone quoted reviewed the pages containing their remarks to ensure
accuracy, and many patiently answered our persistent questions about
what lessons from the AIDS Health Services Program continued to be
salient for them, in light of fast-changing events. The project directors,
in particular, were helpful, reviewing all the material pertaining to their
sites, and trying to help us achieve accuracy, balance, and clarity. They
all deserve credit for making the book authentic.

Because many people with AIDS serve in the care and
advocacy for others with the disease, inescapably several of the people
interviewed for this text have since died from AIDS. We recognize how
much their families, lovers, friends, and co-workers must miss them.
The loss of people like these—people who are involved, who seek
improvement, who give of themselves—is everyone's loss.

Victoria D. Weisfeld
Editor

PREFACE

This book tells the story of nine projects in 11 cities across the United States and how they have tried to meet the challenge of AIDS. Sometimes they were readily successful; more often, they had to take one step backward before they could take two forward. But forward they went. The experiences we had as members of the National Advisory Committee to The Robert Wood Johnson Foundation AIDS Health Services Program were remarkably edifying and taught me much about community action and the power of synergy.

For instance, I chaired a site visit to Atlanta to review the initial proposal for funding from a small, relatively new community-based agency known as AID Atlanta. It was evident that this agency was not only tackling a big problem, but also that it would face many complex hurdles in trying to link with the institutional giant, Grady Memorial Hospital, and the long-time community agency, the Visiting Nurse Association. As we visited intermittently and watched AID Atlanta's progress over the years, we saw that these hurdles did indeed loom in their path; but with good will on all sides, they cleared them. More recently, as chair of the National Commission on AIDS, I found myself in Atlanta again, talking with the staff of AID Atlanta. Their progress has been extraordinary, and the community linkages promise to be sturdy as the epidemic's pressures continue to increase.

The AIDS Health Services Program grantees have now reached a number of important crossroads, with the rest of the nation following not far behind. The choices that are made and the response to situations where there is no choice—where their path is predetermined by others—will greatly influence the state of our nation's health enterprise as we approach the 21st century.

As a disease, AIDS has challenged our nation's health care system to a degree that exceeds the stresses caused by any other single medical condition. That is not only because people with HIV-related illnesses need a full range of outpatient as well as in-hospital services, but because many people reach points in their illness when they also need help with aspects of daily living, such as housing, legal assistance, preparation of meals, and transportation, in order to optimize their quality of life. Of course, the same is true about many of our elderly people and others with chronic illnesses. In that sense, the only new thing about AIDS is the virus. But it is the epidemic pressures of AIDS that have revealed how the lifelines—essential links between those who are chronically ill and their communities—are frayed and broken in many places. The need for a continuum of care has never been so well dramatized as it is with HIV disease. The effect is analogous to seeing one's own home through the eyes of a visitor: all the deterioration, the missing pieces, the cracks, and the poorly working parts are suddenly visible.

The epidemic of AIDS and the plague of illicit drug use also have combined to stretch the health care systems of our large cities beyond endurance. In particular, our public hospitals are on the brink of collapse. The National Commission on AIDS has spent the past year visiting around the country, hearing from caregivers and people in need of care, from administrators and volunteer workers, from homeless people, and from good people across this land struggling to make the system work.

These visits made clear that were HIV stopped in its tracks today, we would have our work cut out for us for at least a decade hence. (The upcoming care needs of the overtly ill will further stress our capabilities, and new discoveries of therapeutic drugs and treatments that might delay onset of clinical illness can only place additional pressure on an already-faltering system.) The fact is that the HIV epidemic is moving inexorably into communities of color and into populations where access to health care was marginal in the best of times. Urgent national attention has never been needed more than now. Full implementation of the Ryan White Comprehensive AIDS Resources Emergency (CARE) Act would help provide the care, treatment, and support services now in very short supply.

From the vantage point of medical management, AIDS presents exceptionally complex challenges to health care workers. "Burnout" has loomed as a threat for many dedicated people as they face a disease with cruel and changing manifestations, for which there is no cure and current treatment promises only to delay an inevitable outcome. There has been notable progress in clinical care, and many new therapies offer increasing hope, but not without the hazard of serious side-effects. Progress in increasing the access of people living with AIDS to experimental therapies has brought innovation at the levels of both clinical care and regulation.

We've seen a shocking disinclination to become involved at all in the care of people with HIV. "Risk" is cited as an excuse, but the risk is far lower from HIV than from many other hazards in the health care workplace. Ignorance is offered as another excuse—but the proper response to ignorance on the part of a professional is to learn, not to walk away. With a million young people soon to be in need of care, this distressing failure of professional behavior must be reversed.

The important work of volunteers will be needed throughout the long decade ahead; but they must not be viewed as "free goods," and they and those who train them must be supported and rewarded appropriate to their enormous contribution. Here, in particular, leadership will be helpful, as it is during any state of emergency.

I sometimes fear that the challenges presented by the HIV epidemic have exceeded our national attention span, because of the relatively slow pace of its evolution. Unlike other disasters that sometimes confront our communities, AIDS has unfolded over nearly a decade. Initially its range seemed to be regionally localized, but that was an illusion. By the fall of last year, the magnitude of AIDS-related tragedy and the scope of personal loss suffered across the nation—even during 1989 alone—dwarfed the toll of all the physical disasters of that trouble-prone year.

Thanks to the immediacy of television news, no matter where we lived, we all participated vicariously in the grief and anguish of those directly affected by the San Francisco earthquake and Hurricane Hugo in South Carolina, and the result was a sense of communal American compassion appropriate to tragedy. The reaction to AIDS has been quite the opposite. Each and every day, thousands of Americans grieve in secret over the loss of family members and loved ones to AIDS. I hope our spirit of humanity will soon be rekindled, and these days shall be no more.

From a national perspective, AIDS seems to have become "old news." But the fact is that the advent of AIDS, like Hiroshima, has changed the world forever. In retrospect, it is too bad that there wasn't some distinctive, visible symbol of the change—like a mushroom-shaped cloud—so that people could have looked up and shuddered and made collective plans to prevent any future occurrence. In fact, the disease AIDS is sufficiently dreadful that even a vivid mental image of the physical wastage and loss of talented youth might have sufficed, if one could somehow have imprinted such a picture on the mind of America.

The most awful aspect of the crossroads at hand is that we are now entering a decade in which greatly increasing numbers of Americans of all sorts—rich and poor, men, women, and children—will face the illnesses provoked by HIV. The broad range of ethnicities inherent in American society will intensify the complexity of the challenge to deliver compassionate care and to voice clear warnings to those at risk but not yet infected. How well we meet this challenge will have profound impact on our society as a whole.

The tremendous long-term social and funding problems posed by the HIV epidemic exceed the capacity of communities to solve alone. However, this report demonstrates that at least in 11 US cities, the complexity has often yielded to creativity and zeal, and new collective strength has been achieved through cooperation and determination. These examples will provide important insight and guidance for other communities that will surely face similar challenges in the very near future.

June E. Osborn, MD
Chair, National Commission on AIDS
Chair, National Advisory Committee
      for the AIDS Health Services Program

Chapter 1
RECOGNIZING THE NEED

Passage of the Ryan White Comprehensive AIDS Resources Emergency (CARE) Act of 1990 was the culmination of a long legislative process. It marked the establishment of a number of important principles about services for people infected with the human immunodeficiency virus (HIV).

Long before this specific legislation was introduced in Congress, these principles were being tested in communities nationwide. And, although some advocates contend that the new law has been inadequately funded, the new principles will set the standard for AIDS service programs nationwide. Based on the experience of The Robert Wood Johnson Foundation-funded AIDS Health Services Program, these principles will affect AIDS care for the better in projects supported by the federal government.

These principles stress the importance of:

- ambulatory services that include case management and comprehensive treatment
- inpatient case management services that prevent unnecessary hospitalization
- a comprehensive continuum of care for individuals and families with HIV disease
- comprehensive services that encompass a wide variety of essential health services, plus essential support services, including transportation, attendant services, homemaker services, and benefits advocacy
- family-centered care for infants, children, women, and families with HIV disease, based on a partnership among parents, professionals, and the community
- outreach services, especially in reaching people with HIV disease in rural areas
- public-private partnerships that foster close working relationships among agencies, and

● home and community-based care assuring the continuity of health insurance coverage.

Like the HIV epidemic itself, these principles first gained widespread attention in San Francisco. They were the basis of the "San Francisco model" of AIDS care. Through a series of subsequent demonstrations, the model was proved. This report describes one of these tests.

When the AIDS crisis broke over the United States in the early 1980s, the staff at The Robert Wood Johnson Foundation (RWJF) in Princeton, New Jersey—the country's largest health care philanthropy—began to consider how that institution could respond.

In 1984, AIDS looked like a problem that needed epidemiology, basic research, and public education—none of which the Foundation supported. At that time, AIDS was a fatal disease with a short patient life-span, and it called for palliative care in the short-term and research breakthroughs in the longer term.

Nevertheless, the issue kept surfacing. Staff were in contact with health care experts in San Francisco and learned of the model for caring for AIDS patients that explicitly addressed access, organization, and costs of care—all issues that did come under the Foundation's grantmaking rubric.

Philip R. Lee, MD, director of the Institute for Health Policy Studies at the University of California, San Francisco, School of Medicine, described this model to the staff as follows: It combined out-of-hospital, community-based support services with in-hospital treatment; it cost markedly less than hospital treatment alone; and it was much more in keeping with the needs and desires of patients.

In late 1985, foundation trustees approved funding for a national competitive health services demonstration program based on the San Francisco model, with the 23 US metropolitan areas having the most AIDS cases eligible to apply. Grants would be awarded in up to 10 sites around the country under the program, called the AIDS Health Services Program (AHSP). After a year's time, during which applicants prepared their proposals, site visits were conducted, and a comprehensive review of applications was completed, nine projects serving 11 communities were funded with a total of $17.1 million in November 1986. It is the experience of these 11 communities that is reported in the chapters that follow.

The AHSP was a demonstration of whether and how the San Francisco model could be applied and adapted widely. The 11 communities are very different from one another and even more different from the city in which the model was first developed—as geographically and socioculturally different as Seattle is from South Florida, Nassau County (NY), or Dallas.

Seattle

Between 1970 and 1987, the Seattle-King County population grew about 20 percent, from 1.16 to 1.39 million. The population of the city stood at 512,000 in 1990, 75 percent of which was white and 12 percent black, with the remainder an ethnic and cultural mix of Asian, American Indian, and Alaska Native groups.

An economy that traditionally relies as heavily on lumbering and aerospace as does Seattle's has ridden a roller coaster, but in recent years, it has diversified, increasing both industry and trade with the Orient through the Port of Seattle. In 1990, the unemployment rate in the metropolitan area stood at 3.4 percent.

The city's reputation for clean streets and civic-mindedness is countered by the second highest alcoholism and suicide rates in the United States (after San Francisco) and a high divorce rate. Seattle underwent a bitter fight in the 1970s over desegregation of public schools, with resultant white flight to the suburbs. Growing population has brought congestion and strengthened already strong anti-growth and anti-development sentiments. The median cost of a house in 1989 was $81,000.

By late 1990, an estimated 1,600 King County residents were living with AIDS or serious HIV-related illness, and the number is expected to double by the end of 1993. Case numbers will continue to increase each year into at least the mid-1990s with new cases numbering about 680 during 1990 and almost 900 in 1993. The cumulative number of serious HIV-disease cases in King County from the first reported case in 1982 through the end of 1990 was about 2,500, with a total of more than 950 deaths. By 1994, the cumulative total forecast is 5,000 cases and 1,800 deaths.

King County cases have been primarily male (98 percent), white (89 percent), and between the ages of 20 and 49 (91 percent). Only 2 percent of cases have been in women and less than 1 percent in children under age 14. Eighty-one percent of cases have been in gay or bisexual men and an additional 11 percent in gay or bisexual men who also used intravenous drugs.

Exposure was attributed to intravenous drug use in heterosexual people in 3 percent of cases as of mid-1990. Hemophiliacs and transfusion recipients accounted for about 1 percent each and cases believed to be due to heterosexual transmission for an additional 1 percent.

San Francisco had a high case load and a well organized gay community that provided many of the community-based support services; its combined city-county government minimized problems in intergovernmental relations; news media were sympathetic; it had a competent public health department that could give direction and coordination to the many actors involved; and AIDS efforts had the willing support of then-Mayor Dianne Feinstein.

Not all of the 11 AHSP communities had been similarly blessed. But, it was important to learn whether more US cities could provide the many services needed in something like the San Francisco model. If not, the consequences could be dire, given the exponential growth of the disease and the impending strain on public hospitals and other resources. The foundation program was intended to help cities cope with the epidemic in ways that would reduce some of the pressure on their health care systems, complete the continuum of care, and make services simultaneously less costly and more what people with AIDS themselves desired.

The Center for Gerontology and Health Care Research at Brown University received a foundation grant to do a long-term evaluation of the AHSP, under the direction of Vincent Mor, PhD. This evaluation is examining service utilization patterns, costs of care, client needs, and experiences with services—based in part on patient interviews—as well as the implementation process in the 11 communities.

Meanwhile, the federal government was watching the progress of the AHSP sites. Initially, federal grant money had gone into New York, Miami, San Francisco, and Los Angeles—four cities where the epidemic was well under way.

Florida

There are three AHSP projects in Florida. The Public Health Trust of Dade County operates two of them: in Dade County (metropolitan Miami) and Broward County (Hollywood-

Fort Lauderdale), two of the most populous counties east of the Mississippi River. The third project is funded through a grant to the Comprehensive AIDS Program (CAP) of Palm Beach County, headquartered in West Palm Beach. CAP operates countywide from there and from an outpost in Belle Glade, some 50 miles to the west and even more distant in demography, culture, and economy.

A look at the December 1988 AIDS case loads in these areas shows the emerging profile of Florida's AIDS epidemic. Not only is the percentage of heterosexually transmitted cases well above the national average, but the percentage of women with AIDS is higher as well—dramatically so in western Palm Beach County, where women made up 31 percent of the AIDS case load, compared to 10.4 percent nationwide.

According to a Centers for Disease Control study released in March 1989, although the rate of new AIDS cases was declining in most major cities, it almost doubled in Miami during the preceding year, from 22 to 42 cases per 100,000 residents. In Fort Lauderdale, the rate of new cases rose 42 percent, from 26 to 37 cases per 100,000. In West Palm Beach, it jumped by 50 percent, from 26 to 39.

Starting with Native Indians and followed by early Spanish, Anglo, and African-American settlers, the South Florida area has more recently been settled by Cuban immigrants, Haitians, other Caribbean peoples, Central Americans, "snow-birds," retirees, and other refugees from the north, as well as the groups of Asians that have grown in number since the Vietnam War. These layers upon layers of communities do not add up to a single community; they exist side by side, generally not interacting.

Intergroup relations in South Florida probably are not helped by the high-power economic and population growth of the region and certainly not by the intensity of the drug problem. Although there is vitality, vibrancy, and a growing cosmopolitan aura in and around Miami, there is also the rawness that often accompanies rapid growth.

The AHSP projects directed by the Public Health Trust of Dade County for both Dade (metropolitan Miami) and Broward (Hollywood-Fort Lauderdale) Counties has had to face squarely these various community forces and try to weave strong project networks despite them.

To a considerable degree, Broward County's growth in recent years—a phenomenal 64.2 percent in the 1970s and an additional 12.2 percent from 1980 to 1986—was at the expense of its neighbor, Dade County, which saw many non-Hispanic whites moving northward, as the Cuban population in metropolitan Miami grew. In the 1980 Census, Hispanics accounted for 56 percent of the Dade County population, compared to 4 percent in the Fort Lauderdale area.

Broward's 1987 population of 1.2 million was largely white (86 percent); the non-white population contained 60,000 to 65,000 Haitians.

Dade County had a population in 1987 of almost 1.8 million that was 79 percent white. Its population grew by only 9 percent from 1980 to 1986 and by only 28 percent during the 1970s. In 1989, the _Miami Review_ estimated there were 90,000 Haitians living in Dade County.

Two very different communities on Palm Beach County's opposite edges are served by Florida's third AHSP project. The smaller of them, Belle Glade, is the first rural community in the United States to have a high incidence of AIDS. Belle Glade, a town of 17,000 people in 1988, is dominated by agribusiness. Farm workers, many of them migratory and many of them Haitians, live in poverty. Forty-eight percent of the population is black, but 99 percent of the 245 people in the town's AIDS case load at the end of 1988 were black. Almost a third of the cases were among women.

Fifty miles to the east is West Palm Beach, a handsome city of nearly 75,000 in the coastal region of Palm Beach County, the richest county in Florida and one of the fastest-growing metropolitan areas in the nation. West Palm Beach's population is predominantly white.

In early 1986, Department of Health and Human Services staff had a briefing about the AIDS Health Services Program in Washington, and ultimately, the department supported a program very much like the AHSP in more than 20 cities—including all the AHSP cities—substantially increasing the funds available to the demonstration sites.

The San Francisco model, simple in outline, is difficult in execution: Keep AIDS patients in their own homes for as long as possible by providing them with the full range of health and support services they need; when they do have to be hospitalized, get them out again as soon as possible. What is needed to accomplish this is a comprehensive array of services rarely available for any patient—home nursing care, psychosocial support for patients and their loved ones, housecleaning, shopping, meals prepared at home or delivered there, and transportation—and requiring the coordinated efforts of a wide variety of health care and social services providers. The health and medical care provided, both in the hospital and at home, involves patients and their loved ones to the greatest extent possible and proceeds from the assumption that patients have the central decision-making role in their own illnesses.

To assist with the complex tasks of coordination, communication, and involvement, the San Francisco model relies on individual case managers for people with AIDS, when circumstances warrant. In consultation with clients and health care providers, case managers develop a plan to meet health and other service needs. Case managers then help people obtain these services, whether by helping them keep scheduled appointments or by advocating for the provision of services when and how they are needed. Often case managers find themselves advocating for client needs ranging from medical care to protection of civil rights to housing.

Nassau County

The population of Nassau County (NY) was estimated at just over 1.3 million people in 1990—90 percent of them white—and was the 19th most populous county in the nation.

A relatively affluent area and site of the first major suburban US development after the Second World War—Levittown—Nassau's housing in 1987 was 73 percent houses, less than 2 percent condominiums, and the rest apartments. The median cost of a home was $91,345, based on 1980 Census data inflated to 1989 prices. Nassau County is also an expensive place to rent an apartment, making it desperately short on affordable housing.

At the end of 1987, the Nassau-Suffolk metropolitan area had the 16th highest incidence of AIDS in the country and the highest AIDS rate among suburban Standard Metropolitan Statistical Areas. The county also was experiencing a high incidence of intravenous drug use among its middle-class. By the end of March 1988, 666 AIDS cases had been reported.

Males make up 85 percent of the AIDS cases, but from this statistical point, Nassau County diverges from the typical pattern: Only 41 percent of cases are among male homosexuals or bisexuals; a close 36 percent has occurred among intravenous drug users. Homosexual intravenous drug users represent 5 percent of the total, and "others" make up 18 percent. Some 61 percent of

*cases are in whites; blacks and Hispanics account for 33 percent
and 4 percent, respectively; other racial and ethnic groups for 2
percent.*

The combination of case management, community-based services, and judicious use of in-hospital care appeared to make the San Francisco model more cost-effective than the more typical pattern of AIDS care evolving in other communities in the mid-1980s, which relied heavily on in-hospital care.

From the San Francisco AIDS experience came leadership for the new Program. Mervyn F. Silverman, MD, MPH, San Francisco's public health officer during the early days of the epidemic when the model developed, agreed to serve as program director. The foundation enlisted as his deputy Clifford Morrison, MS, MN, RN, FAAN, who only three years earlier had been instrumental in organizing Ward 5B at San Francisco General Hospital, the AIDS ward that served as the centerpiece of the city's AIDS efforts. Mr. Morrison also helped pioneer the case management system that has come to characterize the San Francisco model. Dr. Lee agreed to chair the Program's National Advisory Committee, which participated in site visits and provided early guidance to the Program. (This post was later assumed by June Osborn, MD.)

Experience has proved that the community dynamics and tensions around AIDS—more than the medical, scientific, or health care issues—have shaped the nine projects. Events since the grants were awarded in November 1986 have shown that, despite how different the communities are, the demands of coping with AIDS are stressful everywhere.

Dallas

*Texas has a history of parsimonious Medicaid, education,
and social services programs. This state climate affects people in
all Texas cities, including those in conservative Dallas who work to
build public and private investment in basic elements of the social
infrastructure, such as public health, welfare, and education. And
it certainly has affected the AHSP project headed by the AIDS
ARMS Network.*

*1986 estimates show the Dallas metropolitan area had
about one million residents; in the 1980 Census, Dallas's population was 61 percent white, 29 percent black, and 12 percent
Hispanic.*

As of January 1989, there were 1,459 reported AIDS cases in Dallas, 98 percent of them male. Of these, 85 percent were white, 10 percent were black, and 5 percent were Hispanic. Compared to the local population, whites are overrepresented and minorities underrepresented among AIDS patients. Male-to-male sexual contact accounted for 81 percent of cases; intravenous drug use was responsible for under 3 percent. Local estimates put the number of HIV-positive individuals in Dallas County at 28,000 in mid-1988, and epidemiologists projected that the epidemic would not hit its peak there until 1991.

Grantees and Metropolitan Areas Served Under the RWJF AIDS Health Services Program

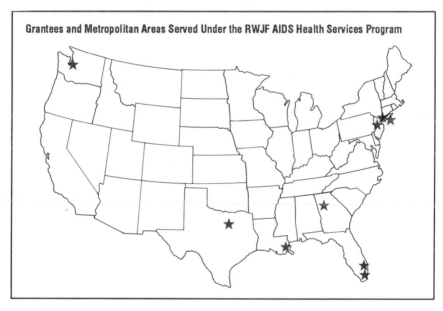

Grantee	Service Area
AID Atlanta, Inc.	Atlanta, Georgia
AIDS ARMS Network, Inc.	Dallas, Texas
Associated Catholic Charities of New Orleans	New Orleans, Louisiana
Comprehensive AIDS Program of Palm Beach County, Inc.	Palm Beach County, Florida
Health Research, Inc.	New York, New York
Nassau County Medical Center	Nassau County (Long Island), New York
New Jersey State Department of Health	Jersey City, New Jersey
	Newark, New Jersey
Public Health Trust of Dade County	Dade County (Miami area), Florida
	Broward County (Hollywood/Fort Lauderdale area), Florida
Seattle-King County Department of Public Health	Seattle, Washington

Nevertheless, AHSP grantees have obtained a wide range of partners that, presumably, make for project success: hospitals, health departments, both traditional community-based organizations and new untried ones, and state and federal government. This wide participation has amplified the credibility with which a small group of people, working in 11 communities scattered across the country, can speak to their counterparts nationwide.

Now ending their fifth year of operation, the people involved in these 11 AHSP sites have learned enough to begin sharing their experiences with communities just coming to grips with the epidemic. That is the purpose of this report.

Keep in mind that this is a snapshot of these projects, with health care providers focusing the lens, at only one point in their development. They—like the AIDS epidemic itself—continue to change rapidly. However, the ongoing implementation of the Ryan White CARE Act makes their message extraordinarily timely, providing new opportunities to apply the fundamental principles of the San Francisco model, as it has been tested and honed in other cities.

Chapter 2
CREATING A
COMMUNITY
CONSORTIUM

THE FIRST STEP: ESTABLISHING NETWORKS

"The big message is that a network must be in place before the project begins, and everybody needs to be involved," says Jane C. Carr, RN, Director, Office of Infectious Disease, Georgia Department of Human Resources in Atlanta.

Atlanta

Atlanta's 1986 population of 421,910 made it the country's 32nd largest city. Continuing the development and expansion that began after World War II, metropolitan Atlanta is the nation's third-fastest growing large metropolis, though the city itself has lost residents to the suburbs. Between 1980 and 1986, the metropolitan area grew nearly 20 percent, to 2.56 million people, while the city of Atlanta shrank by .7 percent.

The city of Atlanta straddles two counties—Fulton and DeKalb—and was 68 percent black in 1980. Of the 18 counties that make up metropolitan Atlanta, all but Fulton are predominantly white. Though unemployment in the region is consistently lower than the national average, so is per capita income. Yet, Atlanta is not an expensive place to live.

The Atlanta AHSP project has been shaped by its location within a gay advocacy group, AID Atlanta. As of June 1988, whites accounted for 74 percent of AID Atlanta's case load, and blacks accounted for 26 percent. Men accounted for 95 percent of the cases. AID Atlanta's case load stood at 581 cases, and 429 people had died of the disease.

That is the first, essential lesson in this compilation of the experiences of AIDS Health Services Program projects. Projects that built strong networks have found that every other person, group, or interest that was involved from the very beginning has multiplied their effectiveness. By contrast, those who start alone in the fight against AIDS will be alone, with only their own resources and support to throw against problems continuously growing in both size and complexity.

Every group has something to contribute: gay people, straight people, whites, blacks, Latinos, the religious community, business, the communications industry, the medical community, all levels of government, public and private service agencies, law enforcement agencies, unions, universities, and political organizations. Whether these groups have money, services, power, influence, time, skills, knowledge, access to people within risk groups, the ability to facilitate a project's operation within the larger community, or the clout to change public or private organizational policies about AIDS, they have resources a project needs.

Breaking down the tendency to deny the importance, or even the presence, of AIDS—which exists to a greater or lesser extent in all communities—is necessary for progress in education, prevention, treatment, and services. People and groups with the ability and influence within their communities to discuss the realities of AIDS in the face of denial are important initial participants in the early networking that precedes a new AIDS services project.

According to Dallas AHSP Project Director and AIDS ARMS Network Executive Director Warren W. ("Buck") Buckingham III:

> Give everybody possible an opportunity to tell you no. Don't deny anybody the opportunity to help. I'm critical of projects that impose limits that are not really there, that assume hatred or homophobia without testing for it. My job is not overcoming homophobia. I am an incrementalist and an evolutionary. I believe that half a loaf is better than none. That's what I've told people to bring to the table, if that is all they have.

Forging alliances with politicians is an early concern for a new consortium. Even if an AHSP consortium had the top-level support of the governor or the mayor—and especially if it didn't—projects found they needed political allies at all levels of government, in both the executive and legislative branches.

Perhaps the ideal way of forging alliances is to involve elected officials in the project's development from the beginning.

In Broward County, People With AIDS Coalition President Michael McCord concludes, "If I were doing this again, I would make sure I had a broader base. We started with five people, all gay white males. It would have made a world of difference if there had been other types of people to reach out to people like themselves in the community."

Typically, AHSP projects that did not start out inclusive were unable to broaden their representation of their own volition. Sometimes they became the objects of hostile takeovers from groups that were not included at the outset. More often, the groups left out formed their own organizations. In some circumstances, competition may be unavoidable and in others even healthy, if it increases accountability, encourages efficiency, and promotes public awareness. However, competition usually produces only negatives, subdividing available monies and other scarce resources and diminishing solidarity. This weakens the project's fund-raising prospects, as well as its advocacy for the needs of people with AIDS, and sometimes it causes fatal delays in getting the message about the dangers of the disease to groups at risk—the worst consequence of all.

The Seattle AHSP project almost excluded some important audiences at the outset. P. Catlin Fullwood, executive director of the People of Color Against AIDS Network, says that the city's minority communities were concerned that they would not be much involved. Ms. Fullwood and other people of color persisted. She explains:

> We wanted a multi-racial coalition, given that we are multi-
> racial in the Pacific Northwest. We didn't want to fragment
> and fight one another over the meager funds available. This
> has allowed the project to have more impact in all of our
> communities. People don't have to forsake their cultural
> identity and racial identity to be a part of this effort.

Don Smith, PhD, chief psychologist of the Georgia Mental Health Institute who has served on the AID Atlanta board of directors since shortly after the group's founding, has reflected on the difficulties AID Atlanta has had establishing a beachhead with groups at risk outside the gay community. He underscores the importance of establishing a broad base: "Otherwise, you will not be able to move, grow, and change with the epidemic. I believe we are dealing with AIDS—not just the gay community. If we are going to ask that others be responsive to us as a community, then we must be responsive to them."

Though in the early days of AIDS, gay men and women faced this disease virtually alone and their efforts to involve others were slow and difficult, second- and third-wave cities, knowing in advance the direction of the epidemic, may have a better chance of avoiding this problem.

THE NEXT STEP: PLANNING

"Clearly, there are real advantages to being a second-wave city," thought Barry Bianchi, board chair of Seattle's Northwest AIDS Foundation. One was the somewhat greater luxury of time that was not available to the cities the epidemic hit so hard, so early. Although Seattle's situation was urgent, "We could look at other cities. We could plan and do strategic thinking."

Indeed, Seattle is a model of planning and foresight. The people involved in the AHSP project there emphasize two key facts: With no cure or preventive technique on the horizon, for purposes of planning, organizing, and acting, AIDS is not going away and will require enormous time, talent, energy, commitment, and money; second, the nation's health care system provides inadequate, yet high-cost care for people with AIDS and does not serve well the growing class of medically indigent Americans.

In fact, the health care "systems problems" encountered in working with AIDS reflect problems that are pervasive, problems that affect the care of all people with serious chronic diseases and progressive disability. Moreover, the demands of AIDS care in many large cities and public hospitals are exacerbating other existing problems having to do with care of people with inadequate health insurance, with no coverage at all, and with few other resources—monetary or social.

Seattle

Method and a devotion to process are characteristics of Seattle, like clean streets, great coffee, and rain. "We can process you to death out here," former mayoral aide Tom Byers says. But, when the process includes all the right people and involves their repeated exposure to the same set of facts over time, its product—consensus about action—is pure gold.

Seattle's AIDS project planning committees began with the construction of a "continuum of care model" that described all the services needed by people with AIDS, the settings in which they would be provided most effectively (home, hospital, community), and specified which needed to be directed by a physician. The number came to 25. Using this list, the planners then inventoried the services available in Seattle-King County. When they were finished, they had a rough idea of which agencies could provide which needed services and, by looking at the blank spots in their matrix, what their yearly work programs would be for each of the four years of the AHSP.

The planners measured the existing capacity of each of the service providers against the need for those services to obtain a reasonably clear idea of what their shortfalls would be in five problem areas: access to services, the limited capacities of volunteer organizations, social services case management, housing and long-term care facilities, and inadequate and poorly coordinated medical care systems.

*This process finally permitted a one-sentence statement of the Seattle AHSP project's mission: While a number of pieces are in place, there is at this time no **system** of care nor a system of providing financial resources to people who need them.*

Together, these facts dictate a strategy of long-term planning and correcting malfunctions in medical care and service delivery at their sources—in laws, regulations, policies, and practices affecting health care organization, financing, and services delivery. As a result, the Northwest AIDS Foundation, using non-RWJF funds, maintains a consultant in the state capital who seeks to organize all Washington cities into a coalition to obtain future funding and programming for AIDS health care and services. And, Seattle's AHSP project maintains a systems analyst to identify blockages in medical and social services delivery so they can be addressed.

A young volunteer in Seattle's Chicken Soup Brigade put the idea in a nutshell: "Set up for the long run from the beginning. Go to agencies that work in gerontology or cancer and find out how they do things. Find out what they are willing to do for people with AIDS, and don't duplicate it. Find gaps and fill them. Don't start over."

The Uses of the Blue-Ribbon Task Force

Politicians often are criticized for ducking a problem by appointing a "blue-ribbon committee" to study it. Yet, in almost every AHSP community that had one, the community task force proved not a way to keep things from happening, but rather a way to get them rolling.

Alan J. Sievert, MD, MPH, director of the Division of Physical Health of the DeKalb County Board of Health, says that when his suburban Atlanta county formed its AIDS task force in 1987, planners deliberately cast their net wide. At the risk of awkwardness, they opted for a membership of 50, drawn from community services agencies, the sheriff's office, the chamber of commerce, Emory University, and AID Atlanta, to name a few. This broad representation lent credibility to task force recommendations.

Likewise, Bill Elsea, MD, MPH, Fulton County health commissioner, believes that Georgia's state AIDS task force played a useful role: "It helped get more people involved to help us with funding and to deflect homophobia," he says. "It also helped get some moderation in the lawmaking area and some consensus on what the policies for dealing with AIDS should be."

- Former Seattle Mayor Charles Royer says his city's AIDS task force "got the corporations involved early—and the private nonprofit service deliverers. People from diverse constituencies were involved, including the gay community." According to Mayor Royer, "That helped us to get a message out that everybody should be involved in this thing and involved from the beginning."
- The Nassau-Suffolk Health Systems Agency, Inc., conducted a bi-county study on AIDS. The agency's report served as the agenda for a first meeting on the subject between the two counties' executives, which led to a plan for a comprehensive response to HIV infection.
- In Dallas, "We deliberately selected a task force of 146 so we could have sufficient numbers of people knowledgeable about each of the areas covered to serve on our various subcommittees," Philip O'Bryan Montgomery, MD, says of that city's AIDS task force, which he chaired. Dr. Montgomery got his work done by dealing through his subcommittee chairs, outlining for them a list of the questions they needed to address. The task force's recommendations, Dr. Montgomery believes, address some fundamental problems with health care organization and financing in Texas.
- In New York City, the task force approach has been used not to create con-

sensus, but to reinforce it. Established by former City Health Commissioner Steven Joseph, MD, this task force was sponsored by the Health Systems Agency of New York City. Advises the task force's director, Glenna Michaels, now a health policy consultant: "Be willing, if you have to, to compromise some substance in your report in exchange for everybody's signing on."

Each of these cities got what it wanted in the way of legitimacy out of its task force: In Atlanta, it was the endorsement of major community institutions; in Seattle, the objective was a blessing from the community; in Nassau, it was the approval of health planning experts; in Dallas, it was a stamp of respectability; and in New York City, it was a badly needed second chance.

New York

In 1988, New York City had a population of 7,352,700, which represents an increase of about 280,000 since 1980. 1990 Census data on the racial composition of the city are not yet available, but 1987 estimates by the Department of City Planning put the proportion of the population that is white (non-Hispanic) at 46 percent, black (non-Hispanic) at 26 percent, Hispanic at 23 percent, and Asian at 5 percent. In 1984, the latest year for which figures are available, 23 percent of the population was below the poverty level. In 1986, the unemployment rate was 7.4 percent. Putting the median cost of a house, last measured in 1980, in terms of 1989 dollars gives an average price of $80,961.

Since the beginning of the HIV epidemic, more than half—52 percent—of AIDS cases in New York City were attributable to male-to-male sexual transmission and 34 percent to intravenous drug use alone. These percentages are changing. The 1989 report of the New York City AIDS Task Force documents that between January and October 1988, the male-to-male portion of the city's new cases of AIDS declined to 41 percent and those in the intravenous drug user (IVDU) risk category rose to over 45 percent.

Clearly, the AIDS/IVDU twin epidemic is in full, costly career in New York City. Mark Kator, executive director of Coler Memorial Hospital, speaking for the task force's Cost Assessment Work Group, reported its best estimate of the costs of AIDS care in the city through 1993 at more than $7 billion. But, as of 1989, eight years into the epidemic, a coherent public strategy had yet to be adopted.

Other recommendations from the New York City AIDS task torce's work groups include these specific items:

- The goal of drug treatment programs should be treatment on demand.
- Education about AIDS should begin in kindergarten and continue through high school.
- State and city government should provide community-based organizations with money and technical assistance to do AIDS education and outreach.
- Neighborhood primary care centers should be established, and where they already exist, they should be encouraged to treat more HIV-infected people on an outpatient basis.
- The federal government should reduce the 24-month Medicare (disability) eligibility waiting period and provide financial assistance to hard-hit cities through block grants.

On the importance of these steps, "We have consensus among the experts and indifference among the political leaders," noted task force member Thomas B. Stoddard, JD, executive director of the Lambda Legal Defense and Education Fund, at a press conference announcing the report's findings.

The reason for continued political inaction in one of the country's more socially progressive states is explained, some say, by New York City's AIDS rates among intravenous drug users and minorities—almost double the rates in the nation as a whole. "Here and in New Jersey and nowhere else," Mr. Stoddard says, "AIDS has become a problem of the poor."

THEN: IMPLEMENTATION STEPS

Locating Power and Responsibility

In the RWJF AIDS Health Services Program, every consortium has a lead agency that is accountable for the project. The choice of that agency in each of the nine funded sites was determined by the applicants. Grantees chose to locate authority and responsibility in an array of different agencies, public and private. Two projects are lodged in state government entities (serving two New Jersey cities and New York City); one in a local health department (Seattle); two in public hospitals (serving Miami/Broward County and Nassau County, NY); two in established nonprofit organizations (New Orleans and, in the beginning, Dallas); and two in community-based organizations (Palm Beach and Atlanta).

When a state entity functions as the lead agency, its broader vantage point can help bring people together, marshal resources, and strengthen coordination through regional approaches. As the lead agency for organizing AHSP activities in Jersey City and Newark, the New Jersey State Department of Health provides project management for multiple sites, primarily through a series of contracts and subcontracts. In New York City, the AIDS Institute of the New York State Department of Health serves as lead agency for administering AHSP activities in a service area that includes all five boroughs of the city and extends into Westchester, Putnam, and Rockland Counties.

Dallas

The lead agency for the Dallas AIDS effort was, almost inevitably, the Community Council of Greater Dallas, a United Way Agency. Former Council Associate Director Buck Buckingham was given the task of directing AIDS ARMS, a community consortium. "We desperately needed the clout and the entree that council sponsorship gave us to get up and running," he says.

The council is a large, well established, nonprofit organization of some 110 community agencies. It provided a ready-made base of organizations to participate in the AIDS consortium, which includes the AIDS Resource Center, Baylor University Medical Center, Chrysalis Home Care and Hospice, the City of Dallas Department of Health and Human Services, the Community Council itself, the Dallas County Health Department, the Dallas Gay Alliance, Dallas Hospice, the Foundation for Human Understanding, Greater Dallas Catholic Homosexuals and Their Families, Oak Lawn Counseling Center, Parkland Memorial Hospital, St. Thomas the Apostle Episcopal Church, the University of Texas Health Science Center at Dallas, and the Visiting Nurse Association of Texas.

Another option for lead agency is a local public health department. The roles and responsibilities of local public health units vary widely across the states. For example, the AHSP project in the Seattle-King County Health Department has made good use of that department's advantages: In 1980, the

Seattle-King County Department of Public Health reorganized, resulting in an agreement that allows the city to identify and fund city health concerns that sometimes are different from those of the county; the department enjoyed former Mayor Royer's political support and benefited from his early leadership in the AIDS area; and, Seattle-King County has an active health and medical research industry.

Alberta Larsen, RN, MN, nurse consultant and advisor in the State of Washington Department of Social and Health Services, was delighted with the Seattle program's origins: "The impetus came from the local level, not the state agency telling local agencies what we could do for them," Ms. Larsen says. Though some first meetings were confrontational, "The most crucial element that evolved from this was mutual trust on the local, state, and federal levels."

The upside of locating the South Florida AIDS Network at Jackson Memorial Hospital, according to the Network's former administrator, Phil Plummer, is the clout that a place like Jackson has. "It provides you with a leg to stand on." Some of the hospital's tangible advantages are: the resources it contributes, its high quality care, and project management. Mr. Plummer, trained as a clinical social worker, also recognizes the downside of a hospital-based project. "Smaller agencies often feel that, when they get involved with an entity as large as Jackson, they have to guard against being gobbled up." These legitimate fears sometimes cause painful power struggles.

A factor in choosing a lead agency is whether an institution is accustomed to being accountable to the wide array of organizations and funding agencies involved in programs like these. A large public hospital like Jackson is already weighed down with daunting internal problems. According to Mr. Plummer:

> People say Jackson doesn't want to deal with AIDS and makes patients sit in emergency rooms for hours. It isn't AIDS: it's the number of patients. Jackson has a 94.8 percent occupancy rate. A bed is barely empty before it is filled again. It is not just the AIDS clinic that has a three- to four-month waiting list. Most specialty clinics do. The hospital is not adequately funded and is not physically big enough. Jackson Hospital has an impossible mission.

Large public hospitals generally are teaching hospitals and, as such, must be responsive to the needs of the medical schools with which they are affiliated. Jackson Memorial depends on the University of Miami for physicians, the university on Jackson for patients. Medical schools have a research— as well as a patient care—mission. As a consequence, patients in teaching hospitals sometimes feel that the institution's priority is not their needs but those of the physician-researcher.

Florida

The organization chart of the South Florida AIDS Network is exceedingly complex. The network operates two different projects in two counties under the sponsorship of the Public Health Trust of Dade County, an entity chartered in only one of those counties to direct Jackson Memorial Hospital, the County's public hospital, and the University of Miami School of Medicine's teaching hospital. One project is in Dade County (Miami), the other in Broward County (principally Hollywood and Fort Lauderdale).

The person responsible for the project day-to-day is the network administrator, who negotiates contracts, coordinates services among providers, monitors the budget, and is responsible for cost effective use of funds and quality assurance. He or she is on the same level as the nursing director, outpatient services director, and administrative director, the latter of whom works for the dean of the medical school and runs the university's comprehensive AIDS program. The network administrator has only an advisory relationship with the network's various service-providing organizations, yet is ultimately responsible for their actions.

An advisory committee works with the president of the trust, the project director, and the network administrator.

In the project, the state and county government units that provide services work shoulder-to-shoulder with private and voluntary service providers; the state by including the regional administrators in the two counties and involving their public health units, the counties by providing social services and involving primary care centers and substance abuse programs.

The Broward project's main medical care providers are Broward General Medical Center, Memorial Hospital of Hollywood, and Northwest Health Center—a state funded and

*directed health center. Both hospitals provide inpatient care, but
Broward General has the heavier case load. Home health care is
provided by a consortium of home health agencies.*

*The principal support service agency is AID Center One,
a volunteer organization that provides transportation, shopping,
companionship, and housing assistance. Also providing transportation, homemaker services, and companionship is Hospice
Care of Broward, Inc. Started in the gay community, AID Center
One has had a minimum of trouble in growing beyond those
boundaries to make good on the phrase that provides its acronym,
Anyone In Distress.*

*The Northwest clinics see symptomatic patients; and four
local primary care centers see only the asymptomatic. Among
them, they had served more than 2,000 people by the fall of 1990,
with a current case load of more than 1,500.*

Bob Parrish, associate director of Grady Memorial Hospital, concurred
in the original decision to place authority and responsibility for the Atlanta
AHSP project in the advocacy group, AID Atlanta. Locating it there, planners
believed, would keep the focus of the project on AIDS, whereas Grady might
lose the project among its universal medical concerns. "That decision failed to
take into account the administrative burden on a little agency," Mr. Parrish says.

Associated Catholic Charities of New Orleans was not a traditional
choice for the lead agency responsibility, given among other things, the tensions
between the Roman Catholic Church and homosexuals. The agency is able to
function in this difficult role in part through the example of Archbishop Philip
M. Hannon (the former head of the Archdiocese of New Orleans), who said
simply that the church has always helped people who are sick. New Orleans
AHSP Project Director Rebecca Lomax, MPH, PhD, says his attitude allowed
everyone else to "keep it simple," too. The project's sponsorship by this key
community agency has helped legitimize its activities in a politically conservative climate.

New Orleans

*A poor city in a poorer state, New Orleans had serious
trouble before the AIDS epidemic came along. According to some
studies, high unemployment and low per-capita income made it the*

nation's poorest large city in the early 1980s. Then the oil econo-
my on which the state depends collapsed, and things got even
worse. The federal government, meanwhile, was dismantling pro-
grams that in the past had cushioned local economies in times of
hardship, programs that New Orleans traditionally relied upon:
public housing, general revenue sharing, and economic develop-
ment assistance. The state government deficit rose to $512 million
in mid-1988. By the fall of 1988, New Orleans's mayor was
proposing a city budget that reduced or eliminated city support
for—among many other things—the police and fire departments,
jails, and the city court system.

Louisiana traditionally has relied on the relatively gener-
ous social programs it inherited from Depression-era Governor
Huey Long to care for a large indigent population, particularly in
matters of health. The system of charity hospitals he fostered is still
in place in parishes throughout the state. However, the state never
has paid for these programs from taxes, instead using income
derived from oil and gas sales.

Although New Orleans's 1988 population of 531,700 was
estimated to be more than 55 percent black, based on the 1980
Census, and local officials say the city is now well over 65 percent
black, its AIDS case load—which accounts for almost 70 percent of
Louisiana's AIDS cases—is 66 percent white. As of December
1990, males accounted for 95 percent of reported cases, and the
principal methods of transmission are male-to-male sexual contact
(78 percent), male-to-male and intravenous drug use (10 percent),
and intravenous drug use (5 percent).

Perhaps the most significant advice of all in deciding where to locate a project's power and authority is to be willing to change the model of organization when events require it. For example, the Dallas AHSP project was initially structured as a project of the Community Council of Greater Dallas, a United Way agency with a solid reputation for attracting influential and dedicated individuals to serve on its board of directors. However, as the need emerged for a coordinated care network to address the complex circumstances of people with AIDS and HIV illnesses in Dallas County, a new organizational structure was created called the AIDS Arms Network. This new organization provides linkages among over 40 agencies.

CHOOSING A BOARD OF DIRECTORS

Choosing board members depends on the functions a consortium expects the board to serve: ownership of a project by all the relevant segments of the larger community and a channel for two-way communication between the project and these groups; the traditional roles of policy-setting, decision-making, fund-raising, and legwork; or support in obtaining "permission" to do the work the project needs to get done.

Bob Parrish's observation, based on the Atlanta experience, may come closest to the realities faced by the first round of cities to take action against AIDS: "When AIDS was not a fit topic for the parlors of 'nice people,' you took whoever would serve on the board. Now there are straight people of some influence in the community who would serve and who do serve. (Their participation) is related to finding continuing funding for the project."

Nancy Paris, chair of the AID Atlanta board in 1989, knows that she was asked to serve because the organization wanted a straight—as well as knowledgeable—person as chair. She had directed the Visiting Nurse Association's Hospice Atlanta, which provided the outpatient health services component of the Atlanta AHSP. "I want people on the AID Atlanta board with good contacts and high profiles in the community. And I want money to be there." She also believes that longtime board members should be willing to let go so others can take their places.

"Organizations are predictable," says Ken South, MDiv, AID Atlanta's director at the time the RWJF grant was made. "If you have a very strong committee that starts things, they hire a weak administrator so they can keep the power. If the group is started by a charismatic individual, he or she picks a compliant board."

Maybe it was inevitable that the first-wave AIDS service programs would be commenced by activist boards, with great potential for conflict with executive directors. Later-wave communities have options. They can choose to invest power in a board of directors to make the principal decisions; or they can choose a strong executive and allocate to the board certain important functions, like raising money and amassing political credibility.

As an example of the latter model, Seattle AHSP Project Director Patricia McInturff, MPA, and her colleagues stopped calling regular meetings of the original AHSP project advisory committee. They did this for two reasons: First, the health department had an existing community-based advisory committee that had been meeting and advising the health department on service issues since 1982; second, the composition of the original advisory committee did not lend itself to dealing with day-to-day project issues. "If something comes up, we get them here with a telephone call," she says.

Board members, alternatively, can be selected for their ability to help with programmatic issues. On Long Island, David E. Jaffe, MPA, AHSP project director and chief operating officer of Nassau County Medical Center, cites this lesson: "We want people of influence who can get us political and community permission to remove obstacles." Often that means involving political people, like the assistant to the Nassau County executive. The county school superintendent was asked to join the board because members believed he could help a project subcontractor go into the public schools with AIDS education. Similarly, "We cut the SSI (disability) application time from more than six weeks down to three by virtue of having a Social Security Administration person on the advisory board," Mr. Jaffe says.

AHSP National Program Director Dr. Mervyn Silverman underscores that "having people representing the communities being served—if not on the board, then certainly in other key roles—is essential."

The pool of people with HIV infection and people who are knowledgeable advocates for them may be expanding. More people with HIV are living longer and healthier, and more professional people with HIV are becoming involved in AIDS-related agencies. In some places, AIDS organizations are choosing as professional administrators people who do not have HIV, and such individuals may make good board or advisory council members. Larry D. Pate, MPA, NHA, the first director of the New Orleans AHSP project, says, "Part of the challenge is not to set aside our objectivity in selecting board members, just because a person has a terminal disease."

Several AHSP projects have provided training in the special skills needed for being an effective board member. One resource for board training is the United Way, which in most communities does it well and will make training available to AIDS health service projects.

Not only board members, but also other allies may need some education. Atlanta's Dr. Elsea emphasizes: "We found that people think they know so much about AIDS when they know so little." For example, some Georgia legislators and executive branch staff were invited to a national seminar on AIDS, and the increase in their knowledge prompted substantial and constructive revisions in a proposed state omnibus AIDS bill.

CHOOSING AN EXECUTIVE DIRECTOR AND STAFF

Often the person who is good at mobilizing a community to invest its resources in an AIDS treatment and services program may not be the person best suited to the day-to-day running of such a program.

Several key attributes are required of project directors: good administrative skills, since funding and support are likely to come from a variety of different sources that need to be kept straight; personnel management skills, to help staff avoid or reduce burnout and to make sure they are interacting well with both clients and the various community agencies involved in the continuum of AIDS care; political skills, to forge strong alliances and a shared understanding of common goals among organizations; and communications skills, since the director is in a good position to be a spokesman to the public not only about the project, but also, if well informed and articulate, on the issue of AIDS in the community.

Florida

Shauna Dunn's success in remedying the organizational problems she inherited as director of the West Palm Beach AHSP project is a tribute to her management skills and leadership:

- She put accessibility of service to clients first and quickly moved project headquarters from a forbidding former prison hospital on the outskirts of town to more inviting headquarters near the neighborhood in which many clients live.
- Her second priority was to mend relationships with the People With AIDS Coalition. They had demanded more consultation and availability; she gave it to them. A more seasoned professional element of the People With AIDS community took control of the coalition, and relationships were soon cordial.
- She next moved on to a complex of staff problems: people who could not give accurate responses to clients' questions; lack of staff understanding of their and the agency's roles; hostility towards clients' ways of living; and, most of all, lack of accountability for staff actions. Between fall 1988 and January 1989, Ms. Dunn replaced most of the staff with experienced professionals and raised salaries commensurately. Accountability she dealt with by following the motto: "Staff respects what management checks."

- *The Belle Glade office staff, which complained of lack of support, information, and attention to their needs, was put under the supervision of an experienced manager who had responsibility for the project's clinical services county-wide. Weekly staff meetings were used to solve problems, provide information, and gather data for planning client services specific to that site.*
- *Finally, Ms. Dunn organized consortia—one of service providers, the other of AIDS educators—to begin attacking the two big problems that still haunt the county: inadequate services for infected children and a lack of education and intervention strategies that will work among Palm Beach County's heterogeneous high-risk groups.*

AID Atlanta's AHSP project has had experience with directors who represented both ends of the management spectrum. According to Dr. Elsea, one director was "good at dealing with people and ideas." The next director was an excellent administrator. Yet, both talents are essential to success, and this project now has a director, Sandra Thurman, who blends the two.

In some cases, two key people can play these roles—an "inside person" who can work with an "outside person." In Seattle, the outside person is Patricia McInturff, who spends a lot of her time keeping a network of agency heads, politicians, community leaders, mayoral staff, and other players informed and interested in the project, while inside, Andy Kruzich kept the project running remarkably smoothly for the two years he was with the project.

In Dallas, Buck Buckingham attempts to do both jobs. He probably spends less time on administration, because he prefers the community outreach role. His staff has tried to share the administrative burden so that he can spend more time in the larger community. Because this outreach is very much needed, Mr. Buckingham recognizes that his efforts need to be supplemented by those of prominent board members.

According to Andy Kruzich, who now directs the New York City AHSP project, the leadership of an AIDS services project needs three key characteristics: a clear sense of the project's mission and goals; an ability to communicate effectively with consortium members; and a good understanding of health care and social service system realities. "It's not the nitty-gritty entitlement details but rather knowledge about the services people with AIDS need that is vital for project leaders," observes Mr. Kruzich.

A project needs to pick staff carefully when it is just getting organized, before one client is seen, believes Sister Anthony Barczykowski, DC, chief executive officer of Associated Catholic Charities of New Orleans. Then it must follow up with ongoing education for staff about AIDS and their attitudes toward the disease and the people affected. "We all have the responsibility to educate ourselves about AIDS. It's here, it's real, it's not going away. We need to talk about the disease so we can help people with it."

A recent college graduate, working as an outreach educator in Belle Glade, said he learned a lot in a hurry about the demands on AIDS project staff:

- "Be culturally sensitive. You have to be able to communicate with people on their level. You have to know what they think."
- "Clients don't assume that you are trying to help them. They assume that they are helping you. And they are, by answering your questions, by giving you information."
- "Don't be too 'textbook' in dealing with drug users. Put all your little idiosyncrasies and biases in your back pocket. They pick up on things like that."

"For people to grow, they have to be able to talk," says Sister Anthony. "We have to be able to listen nonjudgmentally and let them come to their own conclusions."

Chapter 3
MAINTAINING
A CONSORTIUM

Don Smith has thought a great deal about the lessons that come out of AID Atlanta's rocky history. Once a local consortium is up and running, he says, the work of its board has just begun. "AIDS has accelerated the organizational life-span. In normal circumstances, you start with a working board that *is* the organization, then slowly grow to an institutional board. Where it took the Piedmont Arts Festival 30 years to move from one stage to another, it has taken us six."

The rate of change puts demands on board members for flexibility and quick reaction to new circumstances. It demands people who are sufficiently involved to "slave for the agency" but to be able to step aside when the time comes.

Florida

Covering two such disparate sites as Belle Glade and West Palm Beach, Florida, under one project umbrella requires masterful leadership, political skills, management, timing, and luck. For its first two years, the Palm Beach program had virtually none of these except luck. The AHSP project is headed by the Comprehensive AIDS Program (CAP), an agency established specifically to apply for the RWJF grant. One condition of the grant was that the more established Hospice of Palm Beach County administer the project. Hospice had seasoned management but, it turned out, the wrong image and the wrong background for dealing with AIDS.

CAP's first two directors fought an uphill battle, continuously skirmishing with local gay activists. In the fall of 1988,

Shauna Dunn, RN, MS, left her job as an executive in a private psychiatric hospital in Port St. Lucie to become CAP's third executive director. After a joint site visit one month into her tenure, officials from the federal government and RWJF recommended reestablishing a working board of directors for CAP and transferring fiscal and managerial authority for the project to them.

On the positive side, she found strong treatment clinics in both West Palm and Belle Glade, directed by two especially strong doctors and run by the county health department. Other project components include: the Palm Beach County Homes' 19-bed inpatient AIDS wing; the Pantry, a food service for people with AIDS; Hope House; and the Legal Aid Society for help with legal and entitlement problems.

Something else positive that Ms. Dunn found was a favorable image in the heterosexual community. Indeed, this community was far more positive toward the project than was the gay community. The good will such attitudes represent, she saw as literally money in the bank for an organization that must find ways to support itself when Foundation funding ends.

Board members also must be able to help establish good relations with social service agencies, says Dr. Smith. "The best way is to find someone on the inside willing to be associated with you who doesn't bring a lot of extra baggage with them by being organizational mavericks. You can get the mavericks in the organization to deal with you, but they aren't much liked."

INTERAGENCY COOPERATION

Of all the categories in which progress is discernible across the 11 AHSP sites, interagency cooperation is by far the most significant and positive. Even where the lead agency is criticized by various coordinating and contracting agencies, cooperation among the service-providing agencies is clearly evident, and cooperation between them and the lead agency is becoming routine.

The highest degree of interagency cooperation was attained in those projects where someone exerted leadership to enforce it. Nevertheless, even in places where no one had used the power of the purse or of persuasion, and even in places where the project management has been under fire, cooperation could be found—especially at the day-to-day, staff level. The phenomenon is well captured by Sister Anthony Barczykowski of New Orleans, where traditional fragmentation of social and health services in the city and state are exacerbated by severe economic problems, "But, in the case of both the homeless and AIDS, we have been brought closer together," she says.

Changes in procedure can bring about closer cooperation between levels of government, as well as among community agencies. In the Washington State Department of Social and Health Services AIDS Program, Special Projects Coordinator Becky Martelli says, "We operate on the assumption that unless something is written in law, we can make exceptions. If we err, we try to err on the side of the person living with AIDS. We try to have a request for AZT processed in four hours." Rapid processing may not make much difference medically, but Ms. Martelli believes it makes a tremendous difference to the person—it shows someone cares.

Alberta Larsen of the same department says, "AIDS has shone a light on the system and illuminated shortcomings, but it also has demonstrated that the system is more flexible than we think it is." In Washington's case, the system is flexible because state agency representatives have pushed it to be.

Health and social services departments in other states also have been responsive to the needs of people with AIDS and to local health services initiatives.

- Florida's Department of Health and Rehabilitative Services has made its network of county public health clinics available to the projects in Broward, Palm Beach, and Dade Counties and lobbied the legislature for improved funding and one-time initiatives like Broward House, a home for people with AIDS established in Fort Lauderdale.
- New Jersey's Department of Health has responded vigorously to the needs of AIDS patients and has committed funds for prevention of the disease, especially among drug addicts.
- New York and Washington established state-level AIDS institutes or networks to make help available outside their major cities.

Interagency cooperation can mean money for projects. For example, six of eight primary care clinics in Dade County that originally were not included in the care consortium have been brought into it. Three of the eight are elements of city or county government or of the Public Health Trust of Dade County. The remainder are free-standing, not-for-profit federally funded entities. Former Project Director Phil Plummer looks on their participation as one of his big successes, since they bring health care so much closer to people with

AIDS than it had been before. He estimates that these clinics will provide an additional $2 million worth of services annually to people with AIDS and HIV.

Seattle combined the approaches of creating community-based agencies and spinning off to community agencies new responsibilities and money, as they demonstrated they could make the most of them.

Conflict and Cooperation

The chairman of the Metropolitan AIDS Advisory Committee in New Orleans, Conrad Gumbart, MD, has had a standing item on the committee's agenda: conflict. New Orleans Project Director Rebecca Lomax explains why:

> It's difficult to get the organizations in a coalition to put aside
> turf issues. We have groups working together who have no
> historical precedent for working with any other group. We
> are ripe for misunderstandings, mis-communication, rumors.
> The first time Conrad asked us to talk about conflicts, there
> was shock.

But, she believes, his forthrightness has paid off—not by resolving all conflicts, as much as by keeping them from sabotaging the project.

New Orleans

> *The oldest and largest social service agency in the State of
> Louisiana—Associated Catholic Charities of New Orleans—
> administers the New Orleans AHSP. The project and its 12-mem-
> ber consortium are advised by the Metropolitan AIDS Action
> Committee, which is devoted to the coordination of educational ser-
> vices and political responses to the local AIDS epidemic.*
> *The chief provider of medical services is New Orleans
> Charity Hospital, a 700-bed institution that is Louisiana's premier
> public hospital and serves as the point of AIDS referrals for the 11
> other charity hospitals in the state. Charity's C-100 clinic program
> offers inpatient and outpatient care for people with AIDS, and the
> hospital is the only one in the project area that admits uninsured
> patients.*
> *Insured people with AIDS can be admitted to the Tulane*

University Hospital, Southern Baptist Hospital, Touro Infirmary, Ochsner Foundation Hospital, or other local hospitals. Upjohn Health Care Service provides high-tech home health services. Hotel Dieu Hospice offers in-home hospice services. Both are privately owned.

Support services are provided principally by the New Orleans AIDS Task Force (NO/AIDS Task Force) and the Louisiana AIDS Community Network it established. The task force and the community network provide AIDS counseling, HIV testing, a referral service, a buddy program, an AIDS hotline, education, and limited support services to people with AIDS, their families, and significant others.

Case mangement is two-track. The project's case managers handle clients outside of the medical domain; Charity Hospital's case managers are responsible only for medical services while their clients are in the hospital's system. Coordination between the two tracks is a chronic problem. Project Director Rebecca Lomax says that she and a counterpart at the hospital, following the collapse of a formal system of case management coordination, took to doing "paper rounds" over lunch once a month.

As everywhere, housing has been difficult. The one housing program for people with AIDS in metropolitan New Orleans, Project Lazarus, is a seven-bed facility providing room and board for those who are ambulatory.

The State of Louisiana designated 100 nursing home beds for people with AIDS, but given the state's strapped finances, the designation had no practical effect. As in many other jurisdictions, private nursing home operators do not accept AIDS patients.

Her predecessor, Larry D. Pate, believes some conflicts can be prevented by careful crafting of the founding documents of a project. "There have to be clear lines of authority and accountability among service providers and funding sources. Ambiguity in terms of management responsibilities causes problems."

For example, former Atlanta AHSP Project Director Buren Batson says a major lesson he learned is that "it is not appropriate for the administrator of a grant to be a service provider in the same project." His agency, AID Atlanta, has this dual role, which created some confusion along the way. "Grady Hospital does not know when we are talking to them as a partner in our consortium and when we are talking to them as the administrator. And they complain—properly—that we send mixed messages."

Conflict is not always bad. Dick Iacino, MA, deputy director of the University of Miami's Center for Adult Development and Aging, says that Miami AHSP consortium participants have learned two things about conflict: "First, fighting around the same table is better than fighting without communication. Second, you can only coordinate so far. There are times when an agency will just have to compete for funds with another agency in the network." But, competition among consortium members becomes bitter in direct proportion to the scarcity of resources.

"None of us thought when we began that egos, turf, and conflicting motives would play as big a role as they have," Ray Pople, former volunteer coordinator, said of the early days of AID Atlanta. Subsequently, he told community agencies in rural Georgia, to which he provided technical assistance, to anticipate conflict.

Don Smith, too, thinks that having reasonable expectations about conflict helps people deal with it when it comes. "Patience is absolutely crucial. You have to be willing to settle for little increments. Expect things to take a while."

"Consortiums are not as easy as I thought," David Jaffe, who administers the Nassau County AHSP consortium, says. "When you are dealing with multiple organizations, you are dealing with a lot of politics and perceptions over and above those of your own organization."

In a consortium, it is always easier to be the lead agency than a participant who sees problems differently. Mr. Jaffe's consortium meets monthly. "We identify problems in relationships and lay out plans for working them out. We draw up understandings of how things will work from both ends."

Interagency cooperation is, as Larry Pate points out, founded on written agreements negotiated among consortium members. Yet, cooperation has stylistic dimensions, too. In Broward, the style is informal, yet reflects mutual respect among individual organization representatives. As Juliette Love, former director of Center One, says, "We have learned to put all our resources out there on the table so that everybody knows who is doing what. We know each other's priorities. We listen to their issues and address them." In Seattle, the style is not informal but is still highly interactive. A collegial interplay characterizes interactions among the professionals and community health activists who direct the program.

As conceived in 1986, the AHSP project serving New York City residents was designed as a collaborative effort among 20 different agencies working towards the goal of providing "a continuum of care for people with AIDS which links inpatient, ambulatory, and community-based services."

The AIDS Institute of the New York State Department of Health is the lead agency for administering consortium activities and contributes to much of the consortium's overhead (including office space). RWJF funds partially support the consortium's core services and staff, various project-related subcontracts, educational conferences and information materials, and case management consultation services.

After its first year of activity, project leaders identified three major impediments to progress: lack of consensus in decision-making among consortium members; underestimates of the size and scope of staffing required to carry out the project; and resistance to adopting a cross-system approach for case management and data collection. The need for developing a clearly defined structure and establishing patterns of accountability required serious attention.

During 1988, the consortium redefined its mission as being "to identify gaps in AIDS-related services and to coordinate efforts to fill these gaps, with an emphasis on services for people affected by drug use." Interagency coordination was seen as the key.

Several positive structural changes were made, including the reorganization of policymaking functions, from having all 32 consortium members serve on a metropolitan area advisory committee to forming a policy advisory board consisting of 16 representatives of member agencies—four each from city, state, hospital, and community-based agencies. The policy advisory board met monthly (and, later, quarterly) to identify needs, determine program priorities, and develop consortium positions on major issues. A five-member management board was replaced by working groups for specific AIDS-related services. The working groups gather information at the community level, identify gaps in services, conduct educational forums on key issues, and make recommendations to the policy advisory board. The core project staff continues to provide technical assistance to consortium members and other AIDS service providers.

Enforcing Cooperation from Above

Negotiation skills, unambiguous documents, and interpersonal style all are important in the nurturing of an AIDS consortium. When conflicts do occur, it helps to have an overseer with the authority and the willingness to step in to minimize competition and unnecessary conflict.

One such person was former Seattle Mayor Charles Royer. In 1989, he said:

> We won't do business with private nonprofits that won't come together and cooperate. I treat the Human Services Fund (a co-mingling of city general fund money and federal Community Development Block Grant funds) as an incentive. The private nonprofits must come to the city with a plan that shows how they are going to cooperate with other agencies, or they don't get any money from the fund.

In the beginning, the elements of what became the Seattle network— Shanti, the Chicken Soup Brigade, Seattle AIDS Support Group, Northwest AIDS Foundation—were not formally aligned and were competitive. The planning process, undertaken by the Mayor's Task Force on AIDS, made it abundantly clear that people with AIDS would need multiple sources of assistance. In other words, there was more than enough for each organization to do. Moreover, the mayor decreed that there would be only one applicant for AIDS program funding: the health department.

Another such person is Jasmin Shirley Moore, MSPH, who leads the Broward County project. She frowns on competition, particularly competition for money, and she backs up her displeasure with action. "The consortium can discourage duplication of services," she says. "We are trying to convince people to fill needs that are not being met, so we simply don't make referrals to agencies that duplicate."

Fostering Interagency Cooperation at the Personal Level

Pat Campagna, housing and social services coordinator for the Long Island Association for AIDS Care, Inc. (LIAAC), says, "It's really important to be diplomatic with other agencies, to understand that they have budgetary constraints. To some extent, biting your tongue is part of the job."

If she has a problem getting services from an agency, "I always go to the first-line worker first, never to the top," she says. "I have to have a good relationship with these people and not play the aggressive advocate from the beginning. If I have to play that role later on, that's a different story."

Agency bureaucrats are much like other people when it comes to the controversial subject of AIDS, Campagna says. "Attitudes towards people with AIDS vary from office to office. In some offices with strong management that has taken a position and enforced it, staff are no longer fearful or ignorant about the disease. In offices with less strong management, I find the most problems with attitudes."

According to Dr. Mervyn Silverman, "Projects need a formalized setting that accommodates changes in personalities. Organization is the key." While strong, cooperative personalities initially may compensate for organizational weaknesses, if these weaknesses are not corrected, eventually even the strongest, most cooperative personalities cannot paper over the organizational problems.

Seattle

Seattle's AIDS Prevention Project, of which the AHSP project is a key part, is the glue that holds together and augments an array of services to people living with AIDS. These services are provided by more than 15 local public and private organizations. In addition, the project serves as the consortium's data-gathering and planning office. An integral component of the Seattle-King County Health Department, the project provides no direct services, achieving its objectives by working through others.

Most of the inpatient AIDS care is provided by three institutions: Harborview Hospital, the public hospital, takes care of a quarter to a third of people with AIDS; practitioners on staff at Swedish Hospital, the state's largest private hospital, see about 40 percent; and Group Health Cooperative of Puget Sound, one of the country's first health maintenance organizations, sees somewhere between 10 and 15 percent. Other, smaller hospitals in the area also take AIDS patients.

Harborview, the teaching hospital of the University of Washington Medical School, provides outpatient services, supplemented by a small AIDS clinic on the medical campus. Group Health physicians see their AIDS outpatients along with other patients in Group Health clinics, and private physicians on staff at

Swedish see their AIDS outpatients in their own offices.

Support services are provided principally by the Chicken Soup Brigade, Shanti Seattle, and the Seattle AIDS Support Group—all primarily volunteer organizations. Chicken Soup offers practical support (shopping, house cleaning, preparation or delivery of meals, transportation, and other household chores) and attendant care. The other two groups focus on emotional and psychosocial support. Shanti's volunteers offer one-on-one assistance to people with AIDS, their families, and friends. Shanti also trains staff of other community organizations. The Support Group, composed of professionals from mental health and other helping disciplines, offers group therapy. The Support Group runs a drop-in center where people with AIDS can socialize and where various volunteer organizations provide a variety of services—for example, legal help.

The Northwest AIDS Foundation (NWAF) provides these volunteer organizations with administrative support; helps them create systems to recruit, train, and supervise volunteers; and assures the quality of their services. It provides social services case management. It has the responsibility, through a contract with the health department, not only to prepare plans for direct provision of services—including housing—but to raise money to augment existing public and private funds.

NWAF was formed in 1983, after the seventh AIDS death in Seattle, by members of the gay and medical communities. Within a few years, the NWAF board decided to redirect the funds previously used for emergency grants to people in need toward hiring the staff necessary for a really serious organizational commitment.

By 1988-89, NWAF had grown—deliberately and consciously—into a professionally run organization with 30 full-time staff and an annual budget of $2.1 million. Its responsibility in the city's campaign against the epidemic is to coordinate volunteer organizations and directly fill service needs only as a last resort— a lead agency almost, but not quite, equal to the health department itself.

Patricia McInturff acknowledges the subtle but powerful personal relationships in her program. "A lot of informal ties back up the formal ones." Heather Andersen, RN, MN, clinical director of the Hospice of Seattle in the mid-1980s, says, "The referral network that operates now sprang up out of the friendships that developed when we were the only ones seeing AIDS patients."

The young volunteers at the Seattle drop-in center for people with AIDS are more emphatic about the importance of these existing friendships and personal relationships. "We trust them to do what they say they can do," says one. "We don't trust government *per se*; we trust the people in government."

Pat Campagna, the Long Island interagency diplomat, advises people within a consortium to develop relationships with agency personnel—maybe not personal relationships, but ones that are strong enough "so they will call you if they have a problem. I'd call it a reciprocal relationship."

PRIORITIES

AIDS service projects need to set very clear boundaries of what they can and cannot do. For example, Gail Barouh, MA, executive director of the Long Island Association for AIDS Care, Inc. (LIAAC), says her organization "has been approached by government, private agencies, and other groups to do things we don't do: build housing, for one. It was hard to say no, but we believed we would jeopardize our other activities if we agreed." Desirable results sometimes occur: The Huntington Coalition for the Homeless agreed to undertake the housing component because LIAAC consistently refused.

Like Seattle, Long Island doesn't take asymptomatic, HIV-positive people into its case management system. That is a hard limitation to enforce, but even worse, project staff believe, would be to overload the system, weakening it so that it served no one well.

AHSP projects have benefited from periodically assessing specific organizational needs that require special attention. The New York AIDS Consortium has undergone significant changes since its creation, a result of efforts to work with city, state, and community-based entities on joint projects and to design creative approaches to address the complex life circumstances of ethnically diverse people living in a city of over nine million. For example, designing a case management system to work with a set number of individuals in a defined geographic area can't be done without regard for language and lifestyle differences in the population. Such a complicated task has a way of creating its own priorities.

Chapter 4
RUNNING AN
AHSP PROJECT:
SOME ISSUES

Like people with AIDS, organizations that serve them come to think not in terms of being cured of their problems but of developing the skills, patience, and grace to manage them. This chapter reviews a number of key issues they face.

POLITICAL LEADERSHIP

Bill Elsea is one of many Atlantans who are grateful for Michael Lomax's presence on the Fulton County Commission. "He is not the kind of person to hide from problems," Dr. Elsea says. In large part as a result of Commissioner Lomax's leadership, Fulton County was the only one of the three metropolitan Atlanta governments to support AID Atlanta with early dollars.

The money—$40,000 the first year, $60,000 in succeeding years—was important symbolically, as well as financially. It helped to legitimize the agency. It offset an important negative, as well: the image of the agency created by Governor Joe Frank Harris' prohibition of state assistance to it.

Likewise, gay advocate Al Calkins saw changes in the attitudes of politicians in Dallas—changes that ultimately may benefit projects like the AHSP. The gay caucus always has given a candidate for office the choice of publicizing its endorsement of him or her outside the gay community. "In the old days, candidates almost never mentioned our endorsements," he said. "Today, many do. It helps the ones who are in more progressive districts."

AIDS activists, in fact, have made substantial progress in many areas of the country. Members of city councils and county commissioners of surrounding suburban jurisdictions now compete for expressions of support.

Still, there are political difficulties. Georgia legislator Jim Martin represents the Atlanta district that embraces not only the city's gay neighborhoods but also a variety of ethnic groups and conservative Southern Baptists. Says Representative Martin, "AIDS raises the two most politically difficult issues: drug use and sexual behavior."

Atlanta

AID Atlanta, Inc., a community-based volunteer organization formally established in 1984, is the principal AIDS service organization in the metropolitan Atlanta area. The project subcontracts for services with Grady Memorial Hospital, the Visiting Nurses Association of Atlanta, and Hospice Atlanta and offers a variety of direct services ranging from AIDS education and counseling to housing assistance and support services.

The majority of inpatient care is provided through nine area hospitals. The uninsured go to Grady Memorial Hospital, the public hospital that serves as a teaching facility for Emory University Medical School and Morehouse School of Medicine. Grady also offers AIDS outpatient services, as well as limited home hospice care services, the latter in conjunction with the Visiting Nurses Association of Atlanta. Grady's AIDS case load is high.

AID Atlanta's services are provided principally by volunteers trained by the local American Red Cross chapter. Forty percent of AID Atlanta's volunteers are drawn from the straight community. Services include case management, emotional support, practical home support, limited housing, counseling, AIDS education, a buddy program, meals, transportation, housekeeping, and companionship. The Visiting Nurses Association works alongside AID Atlanta volunteers in the provision of some AIDS services.

His track record in the legislature illustrates why AIDS organizations need to comb all levels of the political system for allies and leaders. He and his own allies fended off what could have been very regressive AIDS legislation by arguing that the state should have a five-year plan from the Department of Human Resources before the legislature acted. Bad laws can come about, he believes, simply out of the legislative imperative to "do something" about any important social development.

Representative Martin also helped get a $100,000 appropriation for AID Atlanta through the legislature and past the governor's desk. The sum lifted the governor's proscription against the organization and finally allowed state departments to join its consortium.

Another example of the utility of having state legislators working quietly behind the scenes is Mitch Landrieu, who represents District 90, a New Orleans district that is 55 percent white, 45 percent black, and a mixture of poor and rich. He authored two nuts-and-bolts pieces of legislation helpful to NO (New Orleans) AIDS: expediting Medicaid authorization for AIDS patients and licensing hospices. Representative Landrieu has an unusual way of thinking about his Catholic religion and his efforts to help people with AIDS. "It is a quality-of-life issue to me," he says. "I hope that my reaction would be the same regardless of what kind of disease it was."

Involving people like Representative Landrieu, who are their parties' foot soldiers, pays off in access to higher political leaders. He advised the governor that Louisiana had a problem with paying for AZT. The governor agreed, but said the state could not bear the cost alone, so he personally interceded with then-Secretary of Health and Human Services Otis Bowen for additional funds.

Mitch Landrieu says progress is slow because, as in many places:

> There is a huge anti-homosexual attitude among people in
> Louisiana and, therefore, on the part of the people who repre-
> sent them. What you run into is the attitude that since legis-
> lators themselves don't need social services or public educa-
> tion, they don't have to do anything about these things for
> people who do. So, they will try to do nothing until a disease
> comes along that affects the rich—the movers and shakers.

The prime example of political leadership in the AHSP communities is Charles Royer, former mayor of Seattle. His leadership underscores the necessity of identifying someone—whether elected official or someone else—to apply the power necessary to conduct a calm public dialogue about the epidemic and its lessons for the health care system and to persuade potentially competing organizations to pull together.

*Seattle's former three-term Mayor Charles Royer offers
this advice to mayors in cities just now facing the AIDS crisis: "Get
lucky, and have a tolerant political climate and good corporate
leadership." He then elaborates on his own luck:*

> *Seattle's corporate community responded com-
> passionately and intelligently to the problems of
> their employees. I didn't dig them out. They
> did those things in their companies that they
> needed to do and found their niche outside their
> companies, as well. They were particularly
> helpful in fund-raising, lending legitimacy to
> the efforts of the Northwest AIDS Foundation
> and other groups, both gay and straight.*

*Still, even the most committed corporate leader is no substitute for
the one leader of all the people in the city, the mayor.*

*Mayor Royer understands that his success with his AIDS
programs is due in large part to the tolerant nature of his heterosexual constituents. Not all mayors are as fortunate in this regard.
"There is probably a political cap on people in office and those running for office, a ceiling of tolerance or acceptance you cannot
exceed," he says. "But there is also a floor of decency. Mayors
usually know where these two boundaries are located."*

The former mayor also took a hand in getting state government enlisted in Seattle's AIDS program. Alberta Larsen recalls:

Three years ago, Mayor Royer wrote a letter to the governor
saying that the state was not doing its part. The governor
referred the letter to the Department of Social and Health
Services' long-term care planning group for response. We
asked the Seattle-King County Health Department what they
wanted us to do. We have been meeting for more than two
years now, and what has come out of it, I think, is incredible.

No community organization made the shift from being an organization serving gays to being an organization serving all people with AIDS without some painful soul-searching. "Many in the Atlanta gay community felt let down, as did many nationally, that the development of service agencies has left them behind," former AID Atlanta Executive Director Buren Batson says. But, "We adopted the policy of giving service to anyone who presented himself or herself for service."

Most AHSP partners had made the transition, or were in the process of making it, by the spring of 1989—only to find another painful lesson in store: The groups at risk of HIV infection outside the gay community were not beating down the doors to join them, and what's more, the agencies' efforts to reach out and involve these groups were meeting with little or no success.

In Atlanta, as in many communities nationwide, AIDS has established a beachhead among several population groups that, for one reason or another, steer clear of the community services agencies that the gay men and women who established them still control—or appear to control.

New York

Because of the difficulties of working in so large a city as New York, which has pressing needs for HIV-related services on many fronts, AHSP project staff decided to focus on developing neighborhood demonstration projects to assist families affected by HIV and AIDS. First, the consortium selected three areas in the city with populations between 100,000 and 250,000—East New York in Brooklyn, Central Harlem, and the South Bronx—where HIV risk is significant, and health care resources are scant or poorly coordinated. Then, the consortium identified a lead agency within each of these areas to establish collaborative arrangements with other local AIDS service providers. Each lead agency works with a community-based steering committee to determine major service gaps in the neighborhood, to identify service providers most appropriate to meet these needs, and to assist those service providers in securing federal, state, city, or private resources necessary to implement new programs.

The goal is to provide a continuum of services for HIV-

infected people, including: primary care, hospital care, mental health care, home health services, long-term care, drug treatment services, volunteer services, permanent housing, financial assistance, transportation, counseling and emotional support, and case management.

The East New York Neighborhood Demonstration Project began operation in November 1989, with the New Hope Guild—a local community mental health agency—as lead agency. Program activities are coordinated with assistance from the Brooklyn AIDS Task Force. The project's advisory committee comprises representatives of neighborhood agencies who have been meeting for several years. This committee has selected two priorities for the community: training health care professionals and social service agency staff members to serve people with HIV and AIDS and increasing primary care services. Also, a work group of HIV and AIDS educators was formed that now meets regularly to plan and implement HIV education programs in the community.

Since October 1989, the Central Harlem Neighborhood Demonstration Project has been working to identify HIV-related needs in that community. Serving as the lead agency, the Minority Task Force on AIDS created five work groups involving more than 40 AIDS service provider representatives. These work groups concluded their priority-identification efforts in May 1990, and a steering committee with representatives from each work group is now determining the highest priority needs and ways to address them.

Initiated in October 1989, the South Bronx Neighborhood Demonstration Project has established a steering committee with 21 members, including people with AIDS and representatives from a variety of community agencies. This committee formed three work groups to identify and prioritize community needs. Bronx-Lebanon Hospital is the lead agency. In addition, the project coordinates activities closely with Bronx AIDS Services, Inc., a community-based organization.

Although the neighborhood approach is not a new concept in health care and social service delivery, applying the neighborhood model of coordinated care to AIDS is an innovative effort.

Manuel Laureano-Vega, MD, MS, is a relative newcomer to the AIDS scene in Miami, and his La Liga Contra El SIDA is challenging the primacy of the existing People With AIDS Coalition and of the Miami part of the South Florida AIDS Network by offering Hispanics an alternative to gay-dominated organizations.

"I think the conflict between such groups is inevitable," he says. "It is hard for gay men to let go. That is natural. However, the other at-risk groups have a right to have their own groups represent them. We are demanding that our community give us resources for that representation." Thus, Dr. Laureano-Vega does most of his fund-raising in Miami's increasingly affluent and powerful Cuban community.

The Haitian and black communities don't have the same resources. The outcome in Miami—and other communities where relations among the several AIDS risk groups have become antagonistic—is uncertain. In some communities these antagonisms play out against a backdrop of general political and cultural tensions among ethnic groups. Where such tensions exist, a new AIDS project can anticipate them, because conflict among at-risk groups is not inevitable—it can be stopped before it starts.

In Broward County, the gay community resolved the conflict itself, before it became a major issue, according to Juliette Love, former executive director of Center One, who is black, and Katie Kahrs Sanchez, a former Center One case manager, who is white.

"When I first came to Fort Lauderdale," Ms. Love recalls, "I found some people in the gay community very territorial and defensive about AIDS. When I got into the AIDS arena, I began to see that being defensive and protective of your own can be a good thing."

She says the larger community of Broward doesn't completely turn its face away from the gay community and its AIDS efforts—maybe because it is glad the gay community is taking care of the problem itself, maybe because there were straight volunteers involved in AIDS health services from the beginning, people who had lost friends or loved ones to AIDS and wanted to come to Center One and be helpful.

Two other factors were even more influential, according to Katie Kahrs Sanchez. "The client population changed, and we had to change with it," she says. "And, we decided that we were here to serve all people with AIDS. We made that statement publicly, and we started aggressive outreach."

That decision did not solve all problems. "Some members of the black community hear us, but they don't necessarily come here, for cultural reasons probably," says Ms. Kahrs Sanchez. "They don't want the stigma of coming here, being associated with AIDS, or going to Northwest clinic."

"And some blacks are still in heavy denial," Ms. Love adds.

Another locale that made the transition relatively smoothly is Seattle, where the disease remains largely one of gay white males. Says AHSP Project Director Patricia McInturff:

> Northwest AIDS Foundation was predominantly a white gay organization, but it has changed. Through good leadership, it has become an organization that cares for a larger community and represents the individuals and groups diagnosed with AIDS. It has put more diverse people on its board, changing its original focus. This has been a source of discussion in the gay community, but not a source of great division.

New York City's AIDS Resource Center is another organization that avoided competition. Douglas Dornan, MS, its former executive director, thinks that may have been for two reasons: Heterosexual and bisexual people, people of color, and drug users were involved from the outset, and the organization adopted a mission statement that did not take into account how someone got AIDS. The mission is to provide housing and spiritual and pastoral counseling for people with AIDS. The organization still reflects its largely gay, white origins, yet serves a population that is heavily black and Hispanic.

In New Jersey, intergroup differences are simultaneously acknowledged, accommodated, and ignored. Maria Lebedynec, a case manager at St. Michael's Hospital in Newark, follows the precept that "AIDS is a culturally sensitive disease." She runs two support groups that are distinguished only by the language spoken—English or Spanish. Within each group is a mix of homosexual, bisexual, and heterosexual men, as well as drug users and women. Ms. Lebedynec says the groups were originally integrated this way out of fiscal necessity.

"We were told that this wouldn't work when we started it in 1983," she says. "We have two facilitators in each group, a man and a woman." Ms. Lebedynec is a native Spanish speaker and acts as a bridge between the groups.

Because just throwing people together can be very harmful, Ms. Lebedynec has rules: The groups are closed, and the group itself screens new people for admittance. "I don't want to put people together unless I know who they are and what their agendas are."

Ms. Lebedynec sees more initial tolerance of gay men by drug users than the other way around and says the gays have to be made comfortable in the presence of addicts. She explains:

> The gay men have a great deal to give, and giving it helps
> them overcome any discomfort. We also have made it a rule
> that nobody can come to group unless he or she is sober.
> This makes the gay man feel more comfortable, too. Then
> cohesion sets in, because the focus of the group is on how to
> live with the virus to a full capacity. All group members
> develop understanding and respect for each other's lifestyles.

New Jersey was able to balance the needs of various at-risk groups because its AIDS case load was among the first to be recognized as predominantly drug use-related, project staff believe.

STAFF BURNOUT

Ron Wiewora, MD, MPH, medical director of the Palm Beach County Public Health Unit's AIDS clinics, concedes that emotional burnout is chronic among staff dealing with a disease in which the turnover of both patients and staff is high. In just the first two years of the AHSP, the majority of project director positions had changed hands at least once—some several times. Turnover among other staff was equally high.

Burnout involves physical, emotional, and intellectual exhaustion. It results from constant emotional pressure over a very long period, acting much more like a chronic condition than an acute one. Burnout affects job performance because of its varied symptoms, which include "a general malaise; emotional, physical, and psychological fatigue; feelings of helplessness, hopelessness, and a lack of enthusiasm about work and even life in general," according to research psychologists Ayala Pines and Elliot Aronson. Sadly, individuals who are among the most idealistic and enthusiastic care providers may find themselves in a struggle with burnout.

Individuals working against the HIV epidemic are particularly susceptible to burnout. In addition to meeting the complex demands of growing AIDS case loads with limited resources and fatigue from long workdays, they share three common antecedents of burnout noted by Drs. Pines and Aronson: First, they perform emotionally taxing work that exposes them to their clients' psychological, social, and physical problems; second, they tend to have certain personality characteristics (such as being empathetic and having a genuine desire to help others) that make them vulnerable to the emotional stresses inherent to their profession; and third, they have a "client-centered" orientation that defines the therapeutic relationship between client and care provider as complementary—the professional gives, and the client receives. Under these circumstances, staff morale can erode over time. Consequently, designing and implementing a burnout prevention strategy for AHSP staff has become a serious issue.

An obvious place to start is in developing a solid infrastructure for the organization itself, so that roles and responsibilities are clear. Even—or especially—when coping with an urgent issue like AIDS, a loosely or poorly managed structure creates unnecessary stress. A good structure should include tangible support mechanisms for staff. The first step in preventing staff burnout, says Dr. Wiewora, is to encourage realism: having realistic expectations of what he, as a physician, and other staff can accomplish for clients. Beyond this, there are practical ways of dealing with the problem. The following ideas come from AHSP projects in Palm Beach, Long Island, New Jersey, and Dallas:

- Keep a sense of humor. Dr. Wiewora and his staff often take their cue in this regard from their patients.
- Diversify work assignments. Some projects see that everyone on the team deals with patients and problems that are not related to AIDS; others make sure that line workers have a project they like to do that is different from their principal work.
- Establish reasonable workloads. "Allowing everybody to do everything can only last three years, max," says John Haigney, director of client services at LIAAC. "Then, you must have regular hours and healthy working conditions."
- Offer recognition. Work well done needs acknowledgement, but what is a suitable "bouquet" for one staff member may not be good for another—so personalize, says Andy Kruzich.
- Offer rewards. Good salaries and benefits are needed, underscores LIAAC's Director Gail Barouh, because "You can't spend six to eight months training people who are only going to stay one year. I think my directors are the most important people in this organization, so I put a little more in the pot for them."
- The New Jersey project keeps an eye on the big picture, trying to help staff recognize they are part of something important—beyond the day-to-day

frustrations.

- Hiring staff who are indigenous to the area and familiar with the client population helps, say Steven R. Young, MSPH, director of the New Jersey AHSP project, which serves a predominantly minority, drug-using clientele. "They have to know what they're getting into," he says.

- Schedule time out. The Dallas AHSP project uses regular staff retreats at which staff have opportunities to help guide the future of the organization; it includes twice-monthly clinical supervision of the client services staff to allow them to deal with accumulated grief and stress—called "degriefing"; and it requires that staff take 20 days of annual leave.

- Remember the volunteers. Volunteers need burnout protection, too. Caregivers are notorious for being the last to take care of themselves. Oaklawn Community Services in Dallas requires volunteers to go through bereavement counseling before they can have another buddy.

Bosses can arrange ways to help keep staff from burning out emotionally, but what about themselves? Their visibility makes them a target of criticism. Some are objects of intense political opposition from both the gay and straight communities. When the boss is homosexual, criticism from the gay community can be especially wounding. What do they do to keep well mentally and emotionally?

Buck Buckingham is pleased that his anti-burnout program has worked so well for his staff, but he admits that he had trouble obeying his own rules. "A good two years of six- and seven-day weeks of 20-hour days" got his program up and running. "I don't ever want to do that again." To deal with burnout, he says, "I have become reasonably good at throwing switches—doing things that aren't work-related; going out of town regularly, though these trips often are related to AIDS."

His staff helps. He keeps on his desk a plaque they gave him that reads: "The Buck Doesn't Stop Here Any More."

WORKING WITH THE PHYSICIAN COMMUNITY

Imagination is an important requirement for health professionals dealing with people with AIDS, according to Bill Long, former co-chair of the People With AIDS Coalition in West Palm Beach. "It is most important to identify with the patient and the HIV-positive person, to get a sense from them of what is needed and what needs to be going on." Unfortunately, some health care professionals simply "assume they know what people need, and some of them don't know what they are talking about," he said.

Beyond ignorance about a fast-changing disease, how to treat it, and how to care for the patient with it, is the problem that too few professionals, including physicians, are making the attempt. DeKalb County's public health department sent letters to 1,500 local private practitioners to determine their willingness to treat HIV-positive patients. Eight responded, four of them psychologists.

Ann Collier, MD, medical director of the AIDS clinic at Harborview Medical Center in Seattle, says, "A core of about 10 physicians in the community outside the hospital has been concerned and taken excellent care of people with AIDS. However, there is a very clear economic disincentive to take care of Medicaid AIDS patients. Medicaid pays about 50 cents on the dollar."

Seattle's Swedish Hospital Medical Center surveyed 300 doctors and received 180 responses, 70 of whom said they provide primary care for people with AIDS. However, hospital officials think that most care is provided by only a dozen or so. This is in part because patients want to see doctors who are experienced. Margo Bykonen, RN, AIDS outpatient coordinator at Swedish, says, "I have to talk to patients about the tradeoffs in seeing less experienced doctors who have more time."

MAINSTREAMING THE DISEASE

His long service as a physician in an AIDS clinic has convinced Ron Wiewora that the treatment of people with AIDS must be brought into the hands of the doctors and nurses that treat all other diseases and into the places that they customarily treat them. Individual physicians, he says, will have to learn their limitations in dealing with people with AIDS, just as they do with patients having any number of other complex disorders, and make referrals when necessary to more experienced providers.

Says AHSP Program Director Mervyn Silverman:

> The key is to mainstream but not normalize the response to
> AIDS. AIDS should never be allowed to become a 'normal'
> condition—it simply requires too great and too multifaceted a

response. Plus, unlike the other chronic illnesses you could say the same thing about—like Alzheimer's—you can't forget that AIDS is an infectious disease. Yet today, sadly, AIDS raises relatively little interest and support.

People involved in AHSP projects have a variety of reasons for supporting mainstreaming:

- Lynn Carmichael, director of Jackson Memorial Hospital's innovative visiting physicians program, believes mainstreaming should begin with the very first step. "What I would like to see is family physicians offering anonymous voluntary screening as well as providing services to people who test positive. A lot of the reason for this has to do with confidentiality. Doing it this way puts the HIV-positive person in the setting in which he or she will continue to get services, instead of sending them to a separate screening place."
- Margo Bykonen of Swedish Hospital Medical Center in Seattle has a pragmatic reason for supporting mainstreaming. "I feel that involving more doctors in this will improve the quality of patient care. Some of the doctors that have big AIDS case loads are getting tired."
- Bill Lafferty, MD, an AIDS/HIV epidemiologist, believes, "It's important not to pull AIDS out as the disease of the year, but to use it to arrive at a more comprehensive way of integrating health care to meet the requirements of the human who is ill."

Mainstreaming is a long-term goal. In the short term, warns Clifford Morrison, the risk is that communities may use the "mainstreaming" principle as a smokescreen for not developing any special AIDS services. "If we attempted to mainstream now," he says, "we'd lose everything we have developed."

Philip R. Lee, MD, director of the Institute for Health Policy Studies at the University of California, San Francisco, School of Medicine, explains the need for a comprehensive response to AIDS: "HIV disease presents a whole spectrum of affected people—some of whom are asymptomatic but infected, others who have minor symptoms, and still others with more severe symptoms and a pattern of remissions and relapses." A much broader, more diverse network of doctors and services is needed to take care of this full range of patients. "That is where the private sector response has to be stimulated," Dr. Lee says. "And that is where lessons from the AHSP communities might be of use."

One lesson projects have learned is that doctors need "AIDS 101" training, which should include ways to help patients focus on living, rather than dying. The easiest thing a project can do is to keep community physicians informed of what it is doing. Second, it can involve them in clinical trials at the community level. Third, it can encourage the physician community to develop a program of AIDS Grand Rounds. Many hospitals now hold AIDS Grand Rounds once a month, so that local physicians caring for people with AIDS can get collegial support and so that a broader number of doctors can begin to learn how to take care of AIDS patients. And fourth, it can develop education programs to dispel unfounded fear of contagion among health care workers and promote steps to ensure the safety of the work environment.

The New Jersey Academy of Medicine and the State Health Department have prepared a book entitled "Identification and Management of Asymptomatic HIV-Infected Persons In New Jersey: A Practical Protocol for New Jersey Clinicians" and distributed it to private physicians and other medical care providers statewide. This step-by-step guide offers detailed information about testing individuals for HIV infection and providing appropriate treatment to HIV-infected people who have few, if any, symptoms.

Several years ago, the Long Island AHSP project encountered doctors with a negative attitude about treating people with AIDS. In part through their involvement in the planning of the AHSP project and the networking surrounding service delivery, these attitudes have improved.

Nassau

The Nassau County AIDS Care Consortium (NCACC) is composed of the Nassau County Medical Center (NCMC), the Long Island Association for AIDS Care, Inc. (LIAAC), the Nursing Sisters Home Visiting Services, and the Nassau County Department of Health. The primary goal of NCACC is to develop a coordinated network of health and supportive care services in order to provide continuity of care from hospital to home.

The Nassau County Medical Center, the county's only hospital that accepts patients regardless of their ability to pay, is a 644-bed tertiary care hospital affiliated with the School of Medicine of the State University of New York at Stony Brook. The center has a dedicated 20-bed AIDS unit. The NCMC Intravenous Drug Clinic serves as a diagnostic and treatment center, as well as a site for community hospital referrals. St. Clare's Hospital also has an inpatient unit available to people with AIDS.

> In 1989, the costs of care for 44.4 percent of all dis-
> charges on Long Island for HIV infection and related diseases were
> covered by private insurance, 33.4 percent by public insurance,
> and 22.2 percent of the patients were uninsured.

Michael Baker, MD, acting assistant commissioner for AIDS Program Services of the New York City Department of Health, cites other disincentives. "It must make a difference to you as a doctor if five percent of your patients die as opposed to 40 percent. It is this—as well as the risk of being stigmatized as an 'AIDS doctor'—that keeps some physicians away from AIDS."

"Doctors are into curing, and you can't cure AIDS," says Heather Andersen, now training and curriculum specialist in the University of Washington's AIDS Education and Training Center Program. "That's why I have always thought AIDS is a disease for nursing and social work."

Her former colleague, Susan Kaetz, MPH, believes that the concept of a multidisciplinary approach to AIDS care has not yet taken hold with many doctors. Physicians need encouragement to accept the idea of shared case management, she believes, because it takes away their customary control as the patient's chief manager. "Care of a patient with HIV or AIDS involves more than medical care," she says. "It also involves attention to social, mental health, and family issues."

In an effort to achieve a threshold level of AIDS education among care providers in Florida, the state mandates that they take a continuing education course about AIDS for relicensure. Dick Iacino is one of the trainers:

> The mandated training covers a wide range of subjects, very
> few of them psychosocial. It is not sufficiently flexible to
> allow tailoring to the specific audience. I'm required to give
> physicians material they can get better elsewhere and have to
> neglect attitudinal factors. Physicians can have problems with
> their feelings about HIV and the people it affects. We have to
> help them identify these problems and how they affect the
> care they provide.

Nor is physician education something that, once done, stays done.

ROUND VOLUNTEER, SQUARE HOLE

Volunteers can serve a vital role in meeting the needs of people with AIDS and their families, as well as serving community-based programs in a variety of ways. Volunteers can assist people with AIDS with basic activities of daily living (such as shopping, cooking, cleaning, and paying bills) and help fill the gaps between professional health care services and unmet individual needs. In areas where volunteers cannot be recruited for such tasks, paid staff must be used to provide these services. In addition to providing companionship and direct care services, volunteers can work together with project staff in such areas as fundraising, community education, and special projects.

The value of volunteers participating in AIDS service projects cannot be overestimated. Without the altruistic commitment of volunteers—including Board members and front-line service providers—many community-based AIDS initiatives never would have gotten off the ground.

Although the services of volunteers can be enormously helpful, careful attention must be given to how AHSP projects approach important volunteer management issues. Many sites have designated AHSP staff to be responsible for conducting a thorough screening of volunteer applicants, training volunteers about agency policies and procedures, matching appropriate volunteers to program or client needs, and providing ongoing supervision of volunteer interactions.

When these volunteer management responsibilities are not given enough attention, unnecessary conflicts may disrupt the organization. "Conflicts are an inevitable part of life," said one AIDS volunteer coordinator, "and they happen between volunteers and AIDS agencies."

"For the volunteers to have a good experience, agencies have to be willing to meet their needs. But sometimes volunteers' needs are so in conflict with the aims of the agency that you can't."

A former coordinator of volunteers for Cure AIDS Now in Miami opts for being up-front with volunteers. "Starting a program like this, you have to stress to your volunteers that this requires a commitment, and if they can't manage it, they shouldn't take it on."

A Seattle volunteer agrees. "We try to find a place for the zealots— stacking cans, raising money, or something for which they are qualified other than in-home work."

Another refers volunteers to the agency's mission statement when limits need to be set with a client. "We don't do one-on-one therapy; we do only group work. We don't do transportation. It helps to be able to show people your mission in writing."

Finally, volunteers should not expect to be thanked by the clients. Says a Seattle volunteer:

> Sometimes clients take out their anger and pain on the organization and the person representing it. They must be sure that their rights will be respected, that if they don't like their volunteer, they can say so without being cut off from help. We have worked very hard at soliciting client input to make things better, and we know we have. We volunteers can balance this knowledge against our clients' unhappiness.

Long Island's LIAAC combines volunteer screening with its two-day volunteer training program. Nothing is lost if unsuitable people have experienced the training, according to Kevin Guthrie, director of volunteer services, since "it also serves as community education and disease prevention. A lot of people in at-risk groups volunteer."

However, not all volunteer recruitment efforts are successful. Generally speaking, the New York AIDS Consortium has had a difficult time stimulating volunteer programs to serve people with AIDS with a history of intravenous drug use. Very few significant volunteer-driven projects targeted specifically to the needs of this population have taken hold yet anywhere.

Given the high demand for labor-intensive services involved in caring for people with AIDS and their families and the limited resources available, volunteers will remain very important to AHSP projects. They provide a fresh infusion of enthusiasm and energy. Their time and talents are wanted, needed, and appreciated.

Chapter 5
CASE MANAGEMENT: EARLY VIEWS

When the AIDS epidemic first hit San Francisco, only a single municipal acute care hospital was available to care for the vast majority of people with AIDS. Soon the alarming potential impact of AIDS on the existing health care system was recognized, which stimulated a rapid response from citizens to establish a full range of hospital and community-based services, including comprehensive medical, psychological, and social support.

Shortly after San Francisco General Hospital opened its multidisciplinary AIDS outpatient clinic in 1982, efforts were begun to establish an out-of-hospital care referral system for people with AIDS that included: high-technology home health care services, skilled nursing facilities, hospice care, emergency residential facilities, and community-based counseling and support service programs. Volunteers came forward to assist people with AIDS with basic activities of daily living and to help fill the gaps between professional health care services and unmet individual needs.

As the number of people with AIDS and the number of services increased, San Franciscans saw the need for some formal way to bring services and people together. This coordination/managerial role is usually called "case management." But what case management is and how to implement it are questions the various AHSP projects have interpreted differently, based on local circumstances.

WHAT CASE MANAGEMENT IS

AHSP Deputy Director Clifford Morrison finds the following definition of case management provided by an American Nurses Association task force a useful reference point: "Case management is a system of health assessment, planning, service procurement, delivery, coordination, and monitoring through which multiple service needs of clients are met." According to Mr. Morrison, case management (which may also be called care management or coordinated care) may be described simply as a comprehensive, systematic, coordinated, and planned approach to care that allows an individual to be treated and cared for at the most appropriate level, with a higher quality of care, and in the most cost-effective manner.

"The goals of case management (in order of their priority) are: to provide quality care, to enhance the client's quality of life, and to contain costs," Mr. Morrison says. "But this is an evolving concept, in just its early stages. In 10 years it will look different. For now, I see its primary benefits as a management tool—one which requires good data—that can help in planning and developing new resources and in problem-solving." This requires, he believes, that projects evaluate the case management function in order to make sure it is meeting these administrative needs, as well as client ones.

Specifically, case management focuses attention on meeting the needs of people with AIDS in the following areas:
- promoting and developing out-of-hospital services in community-based and home settings
- developing and using appropriate resources in the least restrictive setting, and
- allowing people with AIDS and their loved ones to participate in decision-making concerning their care options.

Case managers ideally assist and advocate for clients as they gain access to and maneuver their way through the complex health care delivery system. They assist clients by clarifying individual options and services available. They involve clients more in decision-making, and this increases client satisfaction. Case managers communicate information and meet regularly with all members of the health care team involved in their clients' care, as well as keep records of various interventions. Through this all-encompassing approach, an individualized plan is developed, and care is coordinated from a central place, typically based in the community. "It's the three C's," says Mr. Morrison. "Coordination, cooperation, and communication."

IMPLEMENTING CASE MANAGEMENT

Putting effective case management services in place for people with AIDS presents formidable challenges. In the AHSP projects, an evaluation conducted by Vincent Mor of Brown University has shown that these obstacles include:

- adapting community-based case management to the different needs and demands of people engaging in different risk behavior
- providing effective case management in the context of a burgeoning case load and severely limited staff budgets
- coordinating care, given the erratic course of the disease and the often sudden medical and psychosocial crises that arise in patient care
- meeting community care needs, given the current capacity and unwillingness of many traditional home health agencies and hospices to serve people with AIDS
- developing the necessary range of housing alternatives, and
- sustaining the burden of providing continuity of care through systems that rely heavily on volunteers, particularly for the poor and intravenous drug users.

In addition to confronting these obstacles, AHSP projects have faced other pressing issues, Mr. Morrison notes. First, lacking a standardized definition, case management continues to be defined differently and therefore developed differently in various areas of the country. For example, the decentralized approach to case management used in San Francisco has worked because of specific local features, such as city size, populations affected, local politics, and the public health system. In Newark and Jersey City, a structure for hospital-based case management has been put in place to respond to the needs of an HIV-infected population that consists predominantly of intravenous drug users, who generally first seek health care from hospitals or drug treatment centers. Siting case management services in hospitals helped secure their active participation, which was deemed critical to launching any effective and coordinated HIV initiative in New Jersey.

New Jersey

*Jersey City, New Jersey, had a population of over
217,000 in 1988; this compares with populations of 223,500 and
260,350 in 1980 and 1970. In 1988, Jersey City was the 72nd*

largest city in the United States. In the 1980 Census, the population was 57 percent white, 28 percent black, 4 percent Asian, and 19 percent Hispanic. In 1980, 21 percent of the population had incomes below the federal poverty level, and in 1989, Jersey City's unemployment rate was 7 percent.

Jersey City is the most densely populated municipality in the state. Geographically, it is sandwiched between New York City to the east and Newark to the west, separated from them physically by the Hudson River/Upper New York Bay and Newark Bay, respectively.

Not unlike other urban, industrialized cities across the country, Jersey City can be characterized by its changing population mix, high unemployment and poverty, inadequate housing, high rates of teenage pregnancy and infant mortality, and a shortage of primary care physicians available to serve the indigent. A large population of working poor is neither eligible for public medical assistance nor able to afford private insurance. Jersey City has been designated as a medically underserved area.

Newark, New Jersey, had a population of 313,600 in 1988; and this compares with a population of 329,200 in 1980 and 381,900 in 1970. Newark was the nation's 49th largest city in 1988; and in the 1980 Census, its population was 31 percent white, 58 percent black, 1 percent Asian, and 19 percent Hispanic. In 1980, nearly a third were below the poverty level, and in 1989, the city's unemployment rate was 8.5 percent.

Newark covers an area of 23.5 square miles, one-fourth of which is composed of marsh lands and the airport complex. The city is located 8 miles west of New York City. Newark has been a major urban area and center of manufacturing and transportation/shipping. As with many urban areas in the United States, Newark has seen a dramatic decline in its manufacturing industry, middle class population, per capita income, and health care services. Today, its population is poorer, less mobile, and has a greater need for medical services than at any time in its past.

As of September 1990, there were 1,972 reported cases of AIDS among Newark residents and 1,027 reported cases of AIDS among Jersey City residents. Of these, 66 percent of the AIDS cases in Newark and 62 percent in Jersey City were attributed to intravenous drug use; 13 percent in Newark and 20 percent in Jersey City were attributed to male-to-male sexual contact; 4 percent in Newark and 3 percent in Jersey City were pediatric cases; and 17 percent in Newark and 15 percent in Jersey City were classified as being from other or unknown causes. Some 85 percent of *the AIDS cases in Newark and 51 percent of the AIDS cases in Jersey City were non-Hispanic blacks; 5 percent in Newark and 30 percent in Jersey City were non-Hispanic whites; and 10 percent in Newark and 18 percent in Jersey City were among Hispanics.*

The case management approach encounters considerable resistance by many traditionalists in the health care establishment. Providers and even patients sometimes believe that they must give up control over decision-making; sometimes providers object to changing the focus of care from the acute to the chronic or community-based setting.

The need for a clear definition and an understanding of the benefits of case management is vital: Lack of such understanding made case management a political issue in Dallas's gay community. Early in that AHSP project, some advocates treated case management as a frill that drained money away from people with AIDS. That perception has lessened over time, as case management's benefits have become apparent.

The impetus for many community and health care leaders to embrace case management is their belief that it will immediately reduce health care costs. Although in the long run it should be more cost-effective, initially case management may actually increase costs, if new resources and services need to be developed to meet the full range of needs of people with AIDS. The primary emphasis of case management is on quality of care, with cost containment a secondary goal.

The changing populations affected by HIV-related diseases present new case management challenges. Gay men, generally, have been good candidates for case management, and, so far, it also has proved effective in some situations for families, women, and children—notably in Newark. However, comprehensive case management is more difficult (but not impossible) to develop and implement for intravenous drug users and in rural areas and small communities.

CASE MANAGEMENT'S CONTRIBUTION

The case management model, as applied in the AHSP, appears to offer several benefits in providing care to people with AIDS:
- It ensures that the medical, social, and psychological needs of each patient are monitored, regardless of the different settings where care is rendered.

- It has the perceived potential for identifying alternatives to high-cost hospitalization. Early evidence suggested that San Francisco's community-based system of care resulted in reductions in the length and cost of hospitalization for people with AIDS.
- Improved client satisfaction has been reported when a case management system is in place.
- Adopting a case management approach makes sense, given the complexity of needs of people with AIDS that cross multiple areas of professional expertise, such as health, welfare, housing, and the law.

In the 11 AHSP sites, people are practicing case management, although it is implemented in different ways. Even within a site, the definition sometimes varies from one participating agency to the next. In most sites, a client may have as many case managers as agencies providing services, violating the basic case management concept. In Seattle, a given client has only two case managers—one, a medical case manager, who is usually the physician or home health nurse; the other, a case manager for all other services, provided through the Northwest AIDS Foundation.

The New York AIDS Consortium has created a working group that focuses specifically on case management. Begun in September 1988, this group includes representatives from community-based organizations, the City's Health Resources and Services Administration, and the Visiting Nurse Association. In addition to facilitating open discussion among these individuals, the work group's major accomplishments to date include: contracting with New York University to conduct studies on the composition of case management services provided by community-based organizations and hospitals designated as regional referral centers for people with AIDS; and development of guidelines for case management in community-based organizations.

Seattle

Within Seattle's comprehensive system of service delivery, social case management services are provided by the Northwest AIDS Foundation (seven full-time case managers) and the Harborview Medical Center AIDS Clinic (four full-time case managers). The NWAF also coordinates the provision of case management services by Group Health Cooperative, the fourth largest HMO in the country and medical care provider to one in seven people with HIV infection in King County. All case loads are growing. During the second quarter of 1990, the NWAF and Harborview provided case management for 376 people, and Group Health Cooperative case managers served 56 more.

Ann Collier, medical director of Harborview's AIDS clinic, explains how medical case management works there:

> Our view is that from the day that one is diagnosed HIV positive, he or she should have a medical care provider. If they come to Harborview, they become part of our system and use our services. If they walk into NWAF, they are offered choices of Harborview, private medical providers, or other clinics. If they choose Harborview, they plug into our system; if they make another choice, the client is case managed by NWAF if necessary.

> The number of people in a Harborview AIDS clinic averages a little more than 50 per week. Each of Dr. Collier's four case managers has a case load of 40, plus an additional 10 to 20 short-term assistance clients. She concedes that NWAF's average of 35 to 40 is the standard toward which all case management in the consortium aspires. She adds, "We have the advantage of seeing our patients face to face when they come in. Every time there is a clinic, the case managers are there. Doctors and case managers exchange information constantly."

Where the number of points of entry into the system multiply, with them multiply the number of case managers a client might consult. Such an inefficient and redundant system not only is confusing for clients, but also is hard on service providers. In many AHSP sites, as in Miami, the crush of numbers is overwhelming the case management system, says Betsy Pegelow, RN, MSN, former director of special projects for Dade County's Visiting Nurse Association.

The number of clients coordinated by one case manager varies as well, reveal data collected from AHSP case managers in 1988. For example, the three case managers in Atlanta were each responsible for an average of 142 clients, while in Miami, individual case loads were as high as 200. Case managers in New Orleans, Dallas, and Seattle now average a much more manageable 50, 70, and 40 clients, respectively. Since the initiation of the program, most sites have experienced a sharp increase in clients without a concomitant expansion in staff. For this reason, the case load data above are conservative estimates of the demands placed on these professionals today. Redundancy in case management services is particularly frustrating, given these trends. As a result, the Seattle and Nassau County AHSP projects have chosen to limit case management to symptomatic clients who have no one else to help them.

THE PATIENT CARE TEAM

The US health care system is highly professionalized, with ingrained patterns of communication and status that can work against the team approach fundamental to case management.

Mary G. Boland, RN, MSN, employs a fairly straightforward form of case management at Children's Hospital of New Jersey in Newark, where she directs the AIDS Program: Each client has a team of one nurse and one social worker. Once a week they do "paper rounds"—meetings at which staff and case managers review the records of designated clients—with any health care worker involved with a particular child. "The same group of people follows the child in the inpatient and ambulatory care settings, as well as making home visits. This way they get to know the child and the family. They see them over time, in a variety of situations."

Ms. Boland and her staff appreciate and admire the strengths of the families they work with, many of them grandmothers of HIV-infected children, and apparently it shows. "We have close to a 90 percent compliance rate with our appointments," she says, "and we have never lost a family to follow-up." She is making headway with her effort to encourage a family-focused clinic at Children's Hospital that would serve her young patients' parents, also, and add immeasurably to case management at the family level.

Pat Philbin, RN, AIDS care coordinator for Group Health Cooperative of Puget Sound in Seattle, uses a home-based approach in which neither nursing nor social work predominates. "They need to work real closely together as a team," she believes. "Working together makes an incredible difference. When you don't have that, you lose out."

Ron Wiewora of Palm Beach County believes a necessary precondition to effective case management is getting an agency's staff to work as a team. To get them to that point and keep them there, the person in charge has to give them attention and support. He uses paper rounds for the benefit not only of clients, but for staff as well, to check them for signs of stress. When he finds it, he rotates assignments to non-AIDS tasks, to protect workers against burnout.

The different services various consortia members can provide need to be well understood by case managers or, in the face of high case loads, some services may be underutilized. Bob Ward, MSW, executive director of the North Miami Community Mental Health Center—one of seven mental health service providers in the Dade County consortium—is not certain why his agency receives so few referrals for its psychosocial counseling and education services, though he believes part of the reason may be that doctors and other primary caregivers at Jackson Memorial Hospital don't know about all the services available through the consortium.

Florida

The Broward County project's case management system is controlled by state-funded Northwest Health Center. The system works, Center Director Jasmin Shirley Moore says, when its five case manager positions are filled, which is not often. In early 1989, three of the positions were vacant because the $17,000 annual salary was just too low to attract and keep good people. With an average case load of 100 clients for each case worker in 1990, the Broward County project has 17 telephone lines.

When Dade County's case loads began exploding, case management was almost immediately overwhelmed. That project's case management services reside in Jackson Memorial Hospital, where institutional rigidities are perceived as interfering with coordination and collaboration among service providers. Community agency representatives believe they have no input into decisions about the array of services to be offered a client or the plan of care developed in the hospital. Since all care decisions must go through the case manager, community partners in care cannot communicate directly with one another. "Time is lost," says one such representative.

The fundamental problem is simple: There are 20 case workers at Jackson who share only four telephones. Each carries a case load of at least 40 clients.

Sally Dodds, director of Miami's AIDS Health Crisis Network, points to another reason case management and referrals become skewed to certain agencies: "There is a natural gravitation of people with AIDS toward the AIDS agency, and that is us. They come to us just as people with cerebral palsy go to the cerebral palsy agency." Though many models of case management exist, elements that Ms. Dodds considers essential in AIDS care management are multidisciplinary assessment, care planning, service coordination, and psychological support.

The Miami AHSP involves five of Dade County's primary care clinics, which try to minimize referrals as a deliberate strategy. Says Marjorie Brown, MD, chief of personal medical services for the Dade County Public Health Department, "If you start making a lot of referrals, you are going to lose people through the cracks. We offer as much as we can here just to avoid that."

A MANAGEMENT TOOL

Shauna Dunn used case management first to establish accountability among her staff at the Palm Beach AHSP project. She made existing clinical staff from all disciplines serve as case managers, in charge of a specific number of clients. As vacant positions were filled and more experience gained in determining and meeting client needs, she created a new system of three case management teams, each serving a defined geographic area. Teams are headed by a registered nurse and include a social services case manager; they have access to a nurse's aide and homemaker, as needed. The case manager's role is flexible. When a client is in reasonably good health, the social services case manager can do most of the work; when frequent medical interventions are called for, the case manager becomes something like a traffic manager for the nurse.

Ms. Dunn has had to look to unaccustomed disciplines to find case managers: one is a physician licensed in another country; another has multiple degrees in liberal arts, but years of experience as an emergency medical technician, phlebotomist, and sexually transmitted disease counselor.

Buck Buckingham uses case management to discharge one of his organizational tasks in Dallas—monitoring interagency responsiveness. "Part of the way we do case management is that we have a formal weekly staff meeting among the affiliated agencies. We use these meetings to ask what we should do to make their lives and their clients' lives better. Now we are augmenting that by doing a written survey of both clients and service providers."

AIDS ARMS (which stands for Activating Resources to Mobilize Support) Network has two categories of membership. The first echelon comprises the six agencies that provide services under contract to the agency. The second echelon comprises the 40 affiliates that are asked to provide their services to people with AIDS without reimbursement. They come into the network by agreement and attend the weekly network meetings. "We think of them as problem-solvers," Project Director Buck Buckingham says.

The AIDS ARMS Network is primarily concerned with developing an integrated service delivery system. Because state funding was difficult to obtain, the network developed a service system that revolved around community-based organizations and has served over 500 people with AIDS-related illnesses since its inception.

While medical services may be obtained at a variety of hospitals throughout the network's service area, the majority are provided by Parkland Memorial Hospital—Dallas County's only public hospital—and the Veterans Administration Medical Center. Parkland provides inpatient and outpatient medical services, screening and testing, and related education and counseling.

The three principal non-medical providers in the network are Oaklawn Counseling Center (OCC), the AIDS Resource Center, and the Persons with AIDS Coalition:

- OCC, originally established in 1981 as a comprehensive counseling service for the gay community, now serves non-gays as well. It offers counseling, volunteer services, AIDS information and education, and buddy services. The center also serves as an outpost for a Network case manager.
- The AIDS Resource Center provides food, clothing, money, and AIDS education. It, too, is a case manager outpost.
- The Persons with AIDS Coalition provides free transportation, AIDS education and information, referrals to available services, and case management.

The Network's case management system is first-come, first-served, and current clients have priority. Consequently, the Network does not invest much energy in outreach.

CASE MANAGEMENT AND EPIDEMIOLOGY

Case management must evolve with the changing epidemiology of AIDS. For example, "We are seeing more and more bisexual men come forward with their HIV-infected wives," reports Miami's Dr. Manuel Laureano-Vega, founder and executive director of *La Liga Contra El SIDA, Inc.* He continues:

> Perhaps the men go on to full-blown AIDS, and the wives are asymptomatic and have to care for their husbands and for children who may or may not be symptomatic. You treat those women differently than you treat the significant other in a gay male relationship.
>
> When someone has AIDS, the priorities of the family change. The family system gets totally disrupted and fatigued. The mother stays up 24 hours a day with her sick son. We try to provide them with a comprehensive support system: We bring family members in for individual and group counseling, and we provide outreach workers to act as buffers and sources of reliable information.

Case management for family units may require more time and effort—and be more costly—than for single patients, but it is a growing need. Likewise, case management for intravenous drug users may be more difficult, but they are the future of the epidemic. And, case management for a long-term chronic disease, which HIV infection is rapidly becoming, will require further adaptation of this model service.

Chapter 6

THE CHALLENGE
OF HEALTH-RELATED
SERVICES

AIDS services programs that successfully balance the needs of various client groups face still another feat of balance: determining the right mix among three basic program elements—services, prevention education, and client advocacy. The former is discussed in Chapter 6, the latter two in Chapter 7.

Thomas J. Prendergast, epidemiologist for Orange County, California, told delegates to the Second Annual National AIDS Conference in San Francisco in the fall of 1988 the following story:

> A group of citizens was fishing at the bend in a river when all at once they spied a sizable number of people being swept downstream in the churning waters toward a deadly waterfall. They appeared weak and in danger of drowning. One group of fishermen immediately dove into the river. Each swam to the side of a person in distress, latched on, and with great effort towed him to shore. Resting only briefly to recover breath, these fishermen dove again into the water and rescued another batch of drowning people. Finally, exhausted, they were unable to rescue any more.
>
> A second group of fishermen observed these rescue attempts without making any move to join them. After watching for a while, one of them chopped a long branch off a nearby fallen tree and, with the help of her companions, held it out over the stream so that several people could grab on and be hauled to shore at one time. Repeated use of the branch saved more people than were saved by the first group of fishermen, but, still, people who could not hold on to the branch were swept away.

A lone fisherman who had joined neither of the rescue efforts but had watched intently from the bank, turned on his heel and began walking upstream. "Where are you going?" another fisherman demanded angrily. "Stay and help us."

"I'm going upstream to see who's throwing all those people in the water," responded the man (an epidemiologist at heart, commented Dr. Prendergast).

This tale illustrates the interconnectedness of services, advocacy, and education in an AIDS health services project. People are in immediate need of services, some of which a project can provide with its own resources on its own authority. People are in need of other services that can be gained only through cooperation with other agencies that have the authority and resources to provide them. Projects obtain these services through advocacy; without it, services are limited to what a project can provide with its own resources, which are never enough. But without education, the epidemic cannot be affected at its source and, ultimately, all the services and all the advocacy will go for naught.

SERVICES

The Community Backdrop

Each of the 11 sites in the AHSP offer pretty much the same menu of services. Inpatient care is provided by the participating hospital or hospitals. Outpatient clinics are in some places run by the hospitals, in others by other entities. Home health care is provided by Visiting Nurse Associations or comparable organizations. Homemaking chore services are most often provided by volunteers. Hospice care is provided in-home or in a hospice. Transportation is offered by volunteers in some cases, by project staff in others. Home-delivered meals are almost always volunteer-provided. Legal services, counseling, and psychosocial support for the patient and family, lovers, or friends are provided by a wide array of organizations. Housing is usually, but not always, the responsibility of the largest community-based organization in the coalition. Drug treatment services are lodged in diverse agencies. Financial assistance is drawn primarily from federal, state, and local assistance programs, with the agencies that provide it sometimes, but not always, consortium members. Some of the 11 projects have a small amount of their own funds set aside for clients' emergency financial needs.

Explains Gail Barouh of the Long Island Association for AIDS Care:

> Traditional care organizations don't have hotlines, buddy systems, or fast tracks on benefits. We do. And we are doing fine in terms of services in the AIDS-designated hospitals. We are doing fine with home services. What is missing is the middle piece: adult rehabilitation, nursing homes, day programs, chronic care, occupational, physical, and speech therapy.
>
> The other missing piece is family services. You have to support the family if you expect them to continue to care for their loved one. Arrange for them to have respite care and chore services. Treat the total family. If you have a chance to keep the family intact, take it. You will have to work with everyone—not just the person with AIDS—to avoid housing problems, to avoid warehousing.

Where AHSP projects vary is in the relative adequacy and availability of these services. Every project is dissatisfied with the amount of publicly funded services available, but some face bigger problems than others.

Variations in public assistance programs are outside the immediate control of community AIDS projects. They are not, however, totally outside their influence. Eligibility rules and benefit structures are determined by elected state officials and the program administrators they appoint. Yet only one of the AHSP projects—Seattle—works within a network that has a deliberate plan to influence its state legislature and executive branch in ways that would benefit people with AIDS.

Dire state fiscal constraints, such as those in Georgia, Texas, and Louisiana, pose a serious threat to health care services of all kinds. Claudia Byrnes, MSW, associate executive director of the Community Council of Greater Dallas, puts AIDS in the perspective of her state's overall social services climate: "It's not just AIDS that doesn't get the tax dollars. The state's unwillingness to invest in a social services infrastructure punishes people with AIDS just as it punishes other sick people." The Texas AIDS task force report succeeded in effecting a dramatic increase in the state legislature's funding for AIDS, from $3 million a year to a two-year, $18 million appropriation. Still, the state health department estimates the need at $42 million.

Even in a state like New York, where services are relatively generous, AIDS officials fret about the scarcity of resources—especially for drug users— and they look to the federal government to provide at least some help. New York City's Michael Baker has said, "People will not consciously choose to let substance abusers kill themselves with AIDS. They won't have to. Lack of funding for social programs will do that."

When a community's needs are great and cut across social service systems, the private sector cannot easily fill the gap. Though Dallas prides itself on private-sector initiatives, Bob Moos, a Dallas *Morning News* editorial writer, says, "The heavy-hitters just aren't giving the dollars they used to, because of the state of the economy and because they are getting hit up twice as hard as they were 10 years ago."

Moreover, not all communities have, like Seattle, a rich history of community clinics and a local university renowned for research in sexually transmitted diseases or, like San Francisco, a gay and lesbian community already organized well enough to initiate a community-based services system. Buren Batson says that when he started with AID Atlanta, "There were 86 agencies in the San Francisco Bay area dealing with AIDS, most of them community-based. In Georgia, there was one."

Outreach

One service that projects must consider carefully how to handle is outreach. Many people with HIV and AIDS are never seen by local AIDS service agencies and need outreach services to bring them into appropriate care. In fact, in most AHSP sites, staff estimate that their projects see no more than half the AIDS cases that epidemiologists estimate exist in their locales. Some of the remainder—if they are receiving any outpatient services at all—may be receiving them through private physicians, though in most sites, only a few private physicians are known to be active in treating people with AIDS. People who have traditionally been outside the private medical care world—particularly impoverished drug-abusers—remain so, relying instead on their conventional source of care: the hospital emergency room.

AHSP project staff worry about those left out of the AIDS care system, not only because of their possibly unmet health care needs, but also because of the profound isolation into which some—perhaps many—people with HIV and AIDS retreat. The Palm Beach People With AIDS Coalition uses social events to draw out such people, a tactic that has worked to a degree among gay, white men in Miami and elsewhere.

If outreach is incorporated early into a new consortium's service package, it can help demonstrate the kinds and quantity of unmet needs in the community. This information will help establish criteria for services that will make the best possible use of available resources; improve the match between services needed and services offered; and provide the information the consortium's lead agency needs to inform and educate the community and policymakers about the local impact of AIDS and to advocate for the populations affected.

Outreach, which in most health care programs is not adequately reimbursed, is a staff-intensive activity that is usually assigned a low priority. The Palm Beach program looks to the People With AIDS Coalition for volunteers to do this work. Coalition members, dealing with the demands of their own disease, find it hard to attack the outreach responsibility consistently. Even when volunteers are used to do outreach legwork, they require substantial staff involvement for recruitment and screening, training, supervision, and coordination.

The outreach function is discharged in almost as many different ways as there are communities in the AIDS Health Services Program:

- In Miami, some of it is done by Cure AIDS Now, an independent meals provider whose volunteer drivers are regularly out on the streets among at-risk groups. Socials, sponsored by The Body Positive, contribute, too.
- In Belle Glade, CAP nurses hear of people with the disease and make home visits.
- When a CAP case manager and nurse visit hospitalized AIDS patients, he tells both patients and non-patients about what CAP does and leaves brochures with them so they can tell people they know about the organization.
- Seattle's volunteers in Shanti and the Chicken Soup Brigade build outreach into their daily work.
- In all AHSP communities to varying degrees, private physicians serve as sources of referrals.
- The New York AIDS Consortium funds the People With AIDS Coalition's newsletter, *Newsline*. Issued monthly, with a circulation of over 13,000, this publication informs people with AIDS and AIDS service providers about available services and new treatments. It highlights the personal dimensions

of living with HIV. The People With AIDS Coalition also issues a quarterly publication entitled *SIDAhora* for Spanish-speaking people, with a circulation of 12,000.

Abbott Mason, administrative services coordinator of the Palm Beach AHSP project, advises, "Don't lose touch with the people you are serving. There is no 'us' and 'them.' There is only us."

Housing

A community's overall housing market does not seem to affect the difficulty AHSP projects face in finding housing for people with AIDS. Such housing is just as hard to obtain in New Orleans and Dallas, where economic conditions have made the overall housing market soft, as it is in jammed-tight Long Island. The housing market for the poor and near-poor has been uniformly unfavorable across the 11 sites, regardless of community housing market conditions. Because many people with AIDS become indigent, they find themselves competing for shelter in these highly constricted, low-income housing markets.

Nassau

> Nassau County has an excellent health care delivery system. It owns the largest nursing home in the country, A. Holly Patterson, which has 1,200 beds to which another 200-400 beds are being added. But, A. Holly Patterson does not make any of its beds available to people with AIDS. Nor will any of the private nursing homes on Long Island accept people with AIDS, and only a few of the 20 hospitals do so willingly.
>
> In these circumstances, keeping AIDS patients in their homes would appear to be the best housing strategy, even though it serves the needs of only those in good enough condition to live unattended.
>
> People with AIDS find themselves in the same situation as the homeless: When they lose their homes, they are referred to welfare hotels and motels. Or, they go to the hospital. Both alternatives probably cost taxpayers a great deal more than would the provision of good in-home services, nursing home beds, or congregate facilities. Why has so little happened on the housing front? LIAAC staff have a simple answer: "Politics. It's politics."

Nevertheless, not all sites reacted alike to this problem. After more than two years of pursuing conventional housing options, the Long Island AHSP project had produced a handful of new units for people with AIDS. New York City's private, nonprofit AIDS Resource Center has bypassed public housing programs and has found a mix of private apartments and a group home. The Seattle AHSP project worked to change state regulations to permit funding of adult group homes and negotiated agreements with the public housing authority and private sponsors for additional places. The project has since spun off its housing component to an agency that can concentrate on housing problems exclusively.

Although housing for people with AIDS is, uniformly, the most problematic area of activity for all 11 AHSP projects, New York, Seattle, and Nassau County have made some progress, as the following three cases show.

New York City

Started in 1983, the AIDS Resource Center (ARC) in New York City plunged into housing because neither the city nor the state had done so.

ARC's story is a good illustration of how "ready, fire, aim" problem-solving sometimes works. Before the agency knew exactly what to do about housing people with AIDS, it began collecting money in the only way it knew how, setting up tables every single weekend at Sheridan Square and the Upper West Side with fishbowls for people to put in pocket change. With this money, the organization made $250 grants to people who were hospitalized and needed to scrape together their first month's rent.

Step two was a little more thought out. An Episcopal priest had an empty apartment he was willing to rent to ARC for a person with AIDS. The priest's house was the prototype for one of ARC's two housing strategies, and it now has 40 scattered-site apartments in Manhattan and Brooklyn, each with a confidential address, each chosen to be safe from drug activity. Tenants are placed in neighborhoods where they can develop supportive relationships and connections. In addition to a sublet on the unit, the tenants—who include families with children—receive comprehensive case management and other services ranging from recreation and home health care to mandatory drug treatment for addicts. This housing program is based on maximum self-care, according to former ARC Executive Director Douglas Dornan.

ARC's other housing program is Bailey House, once a hotel that now serves as a group home for 44 formerly homeless people with AIDS. Each resident has a private room and bath. Support services include meals, health monitoring, personal care assistance, an activities program, counseling, nutrition and self-care education, psychosocial support, mandatory substance abuse treatment for those needing it, and pastoral care.

"Our daily cost per person at Bailey House is about $125 a day," Mr. Dornan says. "The average hospital bed in New York City costs $800 a day—minimum."

Seattle

In a comparatively tight housing market, helping people with AIDS keep their own homes or relocate has proved an uphill struggle, but the Northwest AIDS Foundation and the Seattle-King County Department of Public Health put together an array of housing opportunities that included, by spring of 1989, 20 vouchers from the Seattle Housing Authority for publicly assisted housing for terminally ill people (most of it occupied by people with AIDS); 15 slots in other Authority housing; two church-supported houses where patients can live independently; a church-sponsored program of subsidies that helps people remain in their own homes or apartments when they can no longer make mortgage or rent payments; and emergency housing at two apartment buildings. Additionally, the Northwest AIDS Foundation coordinates referrals to Rosehedge, an adult family home for six patients who need on-site nursing care, but not hospitalization.

By exception to policy, the state licensed Community Home Health Care, a nonprofit organization that is the largest home health care organization in King County, to operate a facility for six residents (rather than the usual four). The Division of Medical Assistance and the Aging and Adult Services Administration, both within the the State Department of Social and Health Services, share the cost of this care without violating a cap on state expenditures. The state buys private-duty nursing care from the home, with half the cost reimbursed by the federal government. The daily cost of care for each person living at Rosehedge is $222—far less than if residents had to remain in the hospital.

Housing and long-term care needs will continue to multiply in this region, given Seattle's projection that the number of people living with AIDS will more than triple by 1995. Plans are now under way to develop a 35-bed licensed skilled nursing facility and adult day center for people with AIDS. Scheduled to open in late 1991, this facility will offer subacute care, 24-hour skilled nursing care, respite care, and hospice care to 35 residents, as well as adult day health services to as many as 70 people. More than 30 corporations and foundations, 1,000 individual donors, and various public funding sources have provided financial support to launch this $7.4 million initiative, which has received $1.5 million in program-related investment support from The Robert Wood Johnson Foundation.

Nassau County

The shortage of housing for people with AIDS, compounded by the national shortage of low- and moderate-income housing, is especially evident on Long Island. The county government has made county-owned land available to jurisdictions with zoning powers (in New York State, county governments have none), if they will build affordable housing on it. Further, the Nassau-Suffolk Health Systems Agency, Inc., has been asked to study what the state and private insurance companies could do to enable the counties to house AIDS patients in supervised situations.

In the meantime, LIAAC is trying to persuade Nassau County officials to do what Suffolk County has done: subsidize rent for people with AIDS, over and above what they pay for other public assistance clients.

Despite such progress, none of the AHSP projects had, by mid-1989, found a surefire way to provide the most efficient housing service of all: keeping people with AIDS in the homes they had when they contracted the disease. This is another way of saying that none of the projects had found a way to stave off indigence among its clients.

The universal problem with obtaining housing is money. "There is no funding stream to pay for housing," said Glenna Michaels, former director of the New York City AIDS Task Force, the day after the task force made public its 1989 report. "We have no place to house people except in hospitals. We'll bankrupt them. Yet, some people in this state still don't understand how serious this is."

State and local government regulations also limit housing options. In New York City, a combination of local codes and welfare funding regulations keeps the AIDS Resource Center's group home—Bailey House—from realizing the full amount of public assistance funding to which its residents are entitled. In Dallas, publicly assisted housing is racially segregated and inferior. Most project clients try to avoid it by finding roommates and other ways to stretch their monthly disability payments. Fort Lauderdale put a cap on the number of group facilities permitted—not just group homes for people with AIDS, but nursing homes as well—because city officials believed the community had assumed more than its fair share of such facilities compared to its Broward County neighbors.

Florida law recently was amended to exempt AIDS from the state's prohibition on licensing adult congregate facilities for communicable diseases. There are some 200 congregate facilities in Broward County, Jasmin Shirley Moore says. Yet, as of the fall of 1989, only one of them had taken advantage of the change in law to accept AIDS patients. Broward County began to offer Broward House, a private, non-profit, 52-bed adult congregate living facility devoted to people with HIV infections.

When people with AIDS are no longer able to carry on without assistance, the nearly universal lack of nursing home beds or other supervised shelter available to them makes hospital care the only option, albeit an unwanted and costly one. Nursing homes' unwillingness to accept AIDS patients—compounded by a shortage of nursing home beds in many areas—results primarily from a mixture of fear of the disease and economic disincentives. People with AIDS who cannot pay for nursing home care out-of-pocket (private long-term-care insurance is virtually non-existent for this group) must rely upon Medicaid, which in most states reimburses nursing homes at below-market rates.

Drug Treatment and Rehabilitation

According to AHSP National Program Director Mervyn Silverman, "You can't solve the AIDS problem without first solving the drug problem." Yet, drug treatment is just behind housing among the most important missing services in the 11 AHSP communities. Many communities simply cannot quickly enroll drug addicts who want help into treatment and rehabilitation programs, where AIDS education can occur. And, addicts who don't seek help urgently need effective outreach services to help them make changes in their high-risk behavior for HIV infection.

New Jersey

*The New Jersey State Department of Health (NJSDH)
serves as the lead administrative agency for the AHSP project in*

New Jersey, which operates in two New Jersey cities: Jersey City and Newark.

Grant funds provided by The Robert Wood Johnson Foundation have been used to develop the infrastructure for service delivery to people with AIDS, whereas funds from the NJSDH support direct services to people with AIDS. According to Project Director Steven Young, the Foundation funds are "the glue to hold all services together," enabling service providers to reach out to the HIV-infected population, develop a plan of care for individuals, and organize referral arrangements.

The original plan in 1986 was to address the AIDS-related needs of the populations in both cities through a 50-member Metropolitan Area Advisory Committee. However, the project was reorganized, and, currently, coordination and networking in the two cities is through separate bodies, in order to be more responsive to differing political and community organization issues. The Essex County AIDS Network (serving Newark residents) and the Hudson County AIDS Consortium (serving Jersey City residents) encourage linkages among service providers in their respective areas. They pay particular attention to addressing financial issues at the county level.

One development that benefits both communities has been the formation of a pediatric AIDS committee. Starting as an advisory group to the AHSP initiative, this regional group has taken on a life of its own and has grown to address the needs of children with AIDS statewide. It has published a report that includes program recommendations entitled "Generations In Jeopardy," which deals with a wide range of prevention, medical, and social service delivery issues for children.

In order to coordinate the diverse needs of both the people with HIV infection and the providers that serve them, the project emphasizes flexibility. According to Mr. Young, the people involved in this project also have reaffirmed the value of two other key aspects of organizational planning for AIDS-related work: (1) Task forces need to reflect the demographics of the area served; consequently, the composition of various task forces was diversified to include more blacks, Hispanics, and ex-addicts; and (2) Given that 80 percent of people with AIDS served by the program in Newark and Jersey City are drug users, the involvement of people working at drug treatment centers in networking and planning is critical.

In New Jersey, where only an estimated 10 percent of the IVDU population is in treatment, establishing a Drug Rehabilitation Coupon Program proved effective in reaching addicts either unable or unwilling to pay for heroin detoxification. Although not part of the state health department's AHSP project, the coupon program held considerable promise. Over a four-month period beginning in 1986, trained ex-addict street educators distributed coupons valid for up to 21 days of free heroin detoxification to 970 people. Some 84 percent of the coupons were redeemed by people who were actively using heroin intravenously and had not received any drug treatment in the previous year. Once in treatment, addicts received AIDS education from staff within the first three days. Although highly successful in reaching its target population, the coupon program ended due to lack of continued state funding. (Some similar outreach activities have been continued, in Newark and Jersey City, as part of Health Behavior Projects funded by the National Institute on Drug Abuse.)

Overwhelmingly, AHSP projects find that no drug treatment is available in their communities. The shortage in drug treatment is a serious problem that AHSP projects, by themselves, are unable to solve.

Jersey City

In Jersey City—as in Newark and New York City—where the AIDS case load is heavily populated by people who take drugs intravenously, the care plan is simple. Get addicts with AIDS, usually men, into treatment and care as early as possible, which is tough. Look to see whether their spouses and offspring are either HIV-positive or have active AIDS-related disorders. Steer them through a course of care and treatment with a form of case management that has to be especially intense. Activate their families and extended families to be part of their care and support. Help them to die as comfortably as possible.

It is important to be realistic, project officials believe. "For us, a successful case is having someone die with support around them and not out in the streets."

The AIDS case load is between 85 and 98 percent intravenous drug users. Longer life or better quality of life happens, but not for the same reasons as among gay white males. They don't organize into wellness coalitions, but they are very conscientious about follow-up care.

In Jersey City, case managers do a lot of very basic health care with their clients, teaching them how to gain access to the system and how to use it once they do. The case managers have learned they cannot assume that clients know even the most basic things, like what a prescription is and what to do with it. They try to teach people how to manage their lives.

"Nothing will be better for most of these people," a project official says, "and there has to be the possibility of things being better to give a person an incentive to change, to get off drugs. So, what we can do is to make things a little more comfortable."

Their clients are among the most disenfranchised people in the community—a population nobody wants to deal with—and about which staff believe people hold a number of myths:

- *Myth One is that drug abusers are hard to care for. Once in care, their rate of follow-up in Jersey City, at least, is between 85 and 95 percent.*
- *Myth Two is that they are abandoned loners. "They have families and extended families, and this may account for the high rate of follow-up."*
- *Myth Three is that black patients reject care from white caregivers. In Jersey City, they do not.*
- *Myth Four is that the church is the communications link to the black community. "That's only true if you want to link up with elderly black women."*

The New York AIDS Consortium has recognized the need to focus its efforts primarily on those who contracted HIV infection from intravenous drug use for two reasons: (1) the drug-using population has not mobilized to develop support services, as happened within the homosexual community; and (2) AIDS cases among drug users are increasing rapidly, with more new AIDS diagnoses now related to intravenous drug use than to male-to-male sexual activities.

Asked what Broward County could do to improve services for people with AIDS, Katie Kahrs Sanchez responds, "Address its drug problem better. We have one facility that is supposed to handle any Broward patient. It is inundated. There are waiting lists and lines. Even if someone gets in, the drug program cannot medically manage the late stages of AIDS. He can go to jail and get immediate treatment, however."

Drug users are a particularly frustrating clientele. They are difficult to reach; they can be defensive, manipulative, and single-minded in their pursuit of drugs; yet, they frequently are more willing to change their drug-using habits than their sexual practices.

Workers in AHSP projects repeatedly expressed frustration about dealing simultaneously with AIDS and drug addiction. Sister Mary Louise Kelly,
RN, PHN, MSA, former executive director of Nursing Sisters Home Visiting
Service, serving Brooklyn, Nassau, and Suffolk Counties, recounts the frustrations and indignities that drug addicts visited upon her nurses and aides:
clients continuing to use drugs, a client appearing in the doorway naked and
high, a client running out in the street in his underwear "looking for a fix,"
clients exhibiting uncooperative, angry behavior, and clients putting the aides
out of their apartments in unsafe neighborhoods. Some agencies simply do not
admit drug addicts to their service programs, at least not unless they are under
treatment.

Even among care-giving professionals, drug users are clearly consid-
ered the most difficult group in the AIDS population. Yet, those who know the
most about them say over and over, "Treatment works." In many parts of the
country AHSP projects are learning that drug addicts can be reached. Slowly,
painstakingly, they can be helped to change their sexual behavior and manage
their addictions. Treatment is expensive, however, and money is scarce.

Oswaldo Fierro, who directs CURA, a drug treatment and residence
program for Spanish-speaking people in Newark, New Jersey, says, "Treatment
works, and that's a fact. It is expensive. But it works. Which is more expensive: drug treatment or jail?" Though he believes his program can help drug
users, Mr. Fierro says, "There is no room here for people who want to come.
That is the tragedy of it."

Ernest Drucker, PhD, director of the division of community health at
Montefiore Medical Center in New York City, puts it more specifically:

> If you approach addiction in the same way you treat any ill-
> ness and select appropriately among the therapeutic approach-
> es that are available now, then you get a response as good as
> brain surgery or heart valve replacement. The armamentari-
> um is big: acupuncture, methadone, residential and thera-
> peutic communities, day programs, family therapy, anti-
> depressants. Many things will work if you realize that addiction
> is something that needs both medical and social treatment.
>
> When rich people get addicted, they go into treat-
> ment that keeps them earning $2 million a year. But when

poor people try to get services, they encounter these categorical programs that are overbooked, understaffed, undertrained. Yet, if you are serious about treating them, you have to give them more support, not less. It's just like school. A middle-class school can concentrate on being a school. A low-income school has to be a school plus a support system. If you don't spend the $2,000 on support, you have wasted the first $5,000 you spent on treatment.

To deal with the people who cannot give up drugs, even in the face of AIDS, Jack Cox, MA, director of AIDS services for Jersey City's Spectrum Health Care, has changed his expectations. For many years, he worked in methadone programs, which, by tradition, tried to get people to stop using drugs. "Now, because of AIDS, we concentrate on getting people not to use needles. We had to change our program's policy entirely—from terminating people because they did not give up drugs to keeping them for that very reason. Sending them out into a community where there is a HIV seropositivity rate of 50 to 70 percent signs their death warrant."

Mr. Cox also is determined enough to tackle the problem of drug abuse prevention. He and others offer youngsters something that clearly is needed, a program of counseling and help, augmented by a heavy emphasis on sports and physical education. Mr. Cox explains:

The kid who goes out and plays ball two or three hours a day doesn't worry about getting high. But we have deteriorated to the point where kids who go out for sports are ridiculed. The role model is the guy with 17 gold chains around his neck, and sports aren't the ticket out of the ghetto anymore. High schools in the Jersey City area have trouble mustering enough guys to field a football team.

Evolving Service Demands

"With AZT and pentamidine, the average life span of people with AIDS is increasing, and that is changing the way we provide services and the services we provide," Broward's Katie Kahrs Sanchez says. "The emphasis shifts from those services focusing on death and dying to those focusing on living—issues like money management, stress reduction, health maintenance, and maybe even going back to work."

The number of people needing long-term services may expand exponentially, if a trend takes hold to begin treatment earlier—after a positive HIV test, but well before AIDS symptoms develop.

In Broward, Miami, Seattle, Dallas, Atlanta, and Palm Beach, the demand for new kinds of services seems to have been accommodated with relative ease. The same may be said of services to babies with AIDS and their families.

The AHSP projects follow no set process to identify how they need to change their service mix to keep up with the changing nature of the disease. They are so closely attuned to these changes through their clients that, with the glaring exception of being unable to provide adequate services for addicts, they adjust to them quickly. Responding to the needs of new demographic groups is somewhat harder.

Dick Iacino asks:

> Should the service structure in Miami be different, because 45 percent of the population is Hispanic? That might make intuitive sense, but it is probably wrong. Local Hispanics seem to use health services just like everybody else, depending on education and economic resources. This may be different with local Haitians. They may have strong roots in traditional healing practices and may distrust institutionalized health care. They may well subscribe to a very different health belief model.

Serving a variety of population groups calls for flexibility. Mary Boland's pediatric AIDS program at Children's Hospital in Newark has flexibility and—more—a willingness to understand the strengths and the environment of her client families.

Ms. Boland says, in doing so:

> We are learning to market our service to the population so that they will use it. It's not that hard. It has to do with knowing where they are, what they are interested in, and what their priorities are, which are not always my priorities as a nurse. Their lives are incredibly complex, and they have big

issues to deal with like housing, safety, and survival.

There is a lot of suspicion that we are experimenting on their children—usually their grandchildren. It takes a long time to overcome this distrust of institutions. Once they get over it, they open up. The grandmothers are afraid we will be judgmental about how the children got AIDS. We don't push it; through our behavior, we show that it doesn't matter to us how they got the disease."

Special Needs

Several sites have added innovative services to meet clients' special needs. Among the innovations in health care the Nassau County AIDS Care Consortium achieved is the reintroduction of an old idea—home visits by the project's visiting physician to people with AIDS. He hit the road in the summer of 1988 and soon had a case load bigger than he could handle.

The visiting physician was, in part, a response to the facts of life, geography, and infrastructure on Long Island. Long Island starts from the Boroughs of Brooklyn and Queens, extending out into the Atlantic Ocean some 120 miles. A drive from, say, East Meadow in Nassau County past the storied Hamptons to Montauk Point on the Island's tip in Suffolk County can consume an afternoon. Intra-island public transportation is minimal, and the automobile is the vehicle of both choice and necessity. Impoverished AIDS patients often lose their cars or become too weak to drive. Because the Consortium has been unable to provide enough transportation services to meet the need, the visiting physician is one solution.

He also is a partial solution to the problem of case management. The Nassau County Medical Center's case management program emphasizes medical management and discharge planning. The Long Island Association for AIDS Care (LIAAC), by contrast, uses some of its 300 volunteers as case managers for a wide range of nonmedical services. As a result, a person with AIDS is likely to have at least two case managers.

The visiting doctor and the visiting aides from the Nursing Sisters Home Visiting Services see mostly the same patients. The agency tries to schedule aides to visit a patient the same day as the doctor, so they can confer about the patient's condition and needs.

Some other service innovations are:

- In New York City, the People With AIDS Coalition is encouraging services that emphasize living with AIDS. Since a lot of people with AIDS are ready and eager to return to work, the coalition is supporting efforts to teach them office skills or direct them to employers that will accept them.
- The State of New Jersey is replicating the successful pediatric AIDS program developed by Children's Hospital in Newark for the AHSP. A statewide network of five pediatric AIDS programs will be modeled on the Children's program, with Mary Boland and her staff doing the orientation, training, and ongoing support for the new projects. The state is using funds from its federal Health Resources and Services Administration grant to fund the replication.
- In such cases, the value of comprehensive community-based services and family-centered case management is clear. An alternative to hospitalization that caseworkers like is Jackson Memorial Hospital's physician house-call program. It reinforces the patient's ability to remain at home while still receiving good care.
- Another New Jersey effort that could turn into a national model for providing early intervention services or presymptomatic care to HIV-infected people is the Treatment and Assessment Program (TAP). This statewide initiative focuses on health preservation and prevention of HIV transmission, as well as early treatment for people with HIV-related diseases. Five regional TAP centers are located in hospital outpatient clinics and ambulatory care settings in areas where AIDS incidence is moderate or high. The centers provide coordinated, multidisciplinary care, such as administering aerosol pentamidine and other drugs when clinically appropriate, early and comprehensive health status assessments, HIV education and counseling, and ongoing case management. As a result, some 1,500 HIV-infected individuals have had access to a wide range of clinical services—including the opportunity to participate in clinical trials of experimental agents, if appropriate. The centers are full, and several have two-month waiting lists.

A service innovation that provokes different responses is the dedicated AIDS unit in a hospital. Some advocates started out favoring a designated AIDS unit at Grady Hospital in Atlanta, because it seemed to offer the possibility of easier monitoring by volunteers and avoiding isolation, but, according to former volunteer coordinator Ray Pople, "We were counseled to avoid any suggestion of quarantine. I now think hospitalized people with AIDS will be fine as part of the general hospital population."

Says Dr. Bill Elsea of Atlanta, "One thing I regret most is the paranoia the medical community has about AIDS. When you segregate people with AIDS in the hospital, it makes it worse."

Patricia McInturff reports that the Seattle medical community has a very strong bias against a dedicated unit for AIDS. "The philosophy has been that there is no reason to treat people with AIDS differently from people with other diseases."

On Long Island, as in San Francisco, the practice has been otherwise. Steven Levine, MBA, assistant hospital administrator at the Nassau County Medical Center, believes, "A designated ward is good for the support group aspect. Some patients' parents or family come to visit their loved ones and also spend time with the people who don't have visitors."

Chapter 7
TWO OTHER ESSENTIAL SERVICES: PREVENTION EDUCATION AND ADVOCACY

PREVENTION EDUCATION

Although the emphasis on education varies from project to project, education aimed at prevention is one responsibility of grantees in the AHSP. Rebecca Lomax works with a full-time health educator on the staff of NO/AIDS in New Orleans, but that is not the end of education there. "We think of the whole consortium as health educators," she says. "It's almost impossible to disassociate yourself from health education, even if that's not your job title. Even the task force members do health education for legislators and business leaders."

Education—primarily providing information to people at risk of AIDS about how to avoid the disease and the skills they need to prevent it—includes educating various target audiences and the public at large about the disease and the needs of people with AIDS.

Some AHSP projects have spun off their education functions. The Broward AIDS Foundation was set up to educate the business community on the need for funding and for corporate policies and practices to ensure humane treatment of employees with AIDS. The spinoff agency concentrates its work on the education front and frees the people and agencies in the service delivery consortium of one additional task. Likewise, the Seattle AHSP project has delegated education for gay men to the Northwest AIDS Foundation.

Rolando D. Rodriguez, MS, has learned this lesson about education from his experiences raising money for Genesis House in Miami: "to expect people to be people and to react with fear and every other emotion until they learn what the reality of AIDS and having AIDS is. With your persistence, they will come through."

Atlanta

AID Atlanta serves the area within a four-hour drive of the city. Gay and bisexual men and women come to the big city periodically to do the kind of socializing they are unable to do in suburban and rural towns. This at-risk audience, whether within or outside Atlanta, is not necessarily well schooled or very sophisticated. In 1983, clinical, evasive language did not seem indicated for AID Atlanta's educational messages about safer sex. The agency therefore produced a brochure that used the language gay men use and distributed it in the bars, baths, and other gathering places that gay men frequent.

"By and large, the brochure was well received by the population for which it was intended," Don Smith recalls.

But Citizens for Public Awareness, a group lobbying against a gay rights ordinance before the Atlanta City Council, sent a copy of the brochure to every member of the state legislature and to the governor with a letter asking their help in defeating the ordinance. AID Atlanta was still recovering from this public relations disaster six years later. Apparently in response, Governor Harris ordered state officials to have nothing to do with the group and to give it no state funds. From 1983 until 1988, the government of the state with the eighth largest AIDS case load in the nation boycotted the only AIDS health services agency of the state's largest city.

"The word on the grapevine was that the governor didn't even want to hear the word 'AIDS,'" according to Joseph A. Wilber, MD, medical consultant to the Office of Infectious Disease, Georgia Department of Human Resources. When he is not lobbying for the department in the state legislature, Dr. Wilber volunteers at the Grady AIDS clinic and for a local AIDS housing group.

Jane Carr, who is responsible for coordinating all the state government's AIDS programs, says, "That brochure really put us in the ditch for years." She credits the Atlanta gay community for rapidly sizing up the epidemic's severity in Georgia, and she understands why AID Atlanta believed it was right to be explicit. "But in hindsight, it was not right, because it created a climate

*that caused government not to be able to associate with AID
Atlanta publicly. Two years in a row, we included AID Atlanta in
our budget requests, and two years in a row, our requests for all
AIDS funding were denied." Nor could her agency provide much-
needed technical assistance.*

*Buren Batson says he set high priority on getting the gov-
ernor's ban rescinded and AID Atlanta's stock with state government restored after he took over as AID Atlanta's third executive
director in July 1987. "I knew that if we got as little as $1 from the
state government, it would establish a relationship with the state
that would legitimize us."*

*With the help of others both within and outside state gov-
ernment, Mr. Batson worked away quietly on the problem over the
fall and winter of 1987. In 1988, AID Atlanta was appropriated
$100,000 to pay for case management. "The significance of the
appropriation was not just the money," says state representative
Jim Martin. "It was the credibility it conferred on the agency. It
made the governor's proscription null and void."*

Cultural Dimensions of Education

Gay white men have shown that dramatic changes in sexual behavior are possible. The job now is to continue developing education techniques specific to
other groups. While cultural factors may or may not influence the manner in
which health services are provided, Dick Iacino says they almost always power-
fully influence the way education and prevention services should be planned
and delivered.

"Behavior puts you at risk of AIDS," he emphasizes, and reaching people with a prevention message that will influence behavior is heavily affected by
cultural factors. "In New York City, the principal method of infection among
Hispanics is intravenous drug abuse. Here in Miami, the Cuban population
doesn't use needles much. Though both groups are Hispanic, we must focus on
risk behavior rather than ethnicity."

Also in Miami, Dr. Laureano-Vega founded *La Liga Contra El SIDA*, The
League against AIDS, to prevent AIDS among Hispanics. *La Liga* will do what
gay white community organizations did before it, but very differently: "We start
with awareness-raising. We have to make people aware there is an epidemic
threatening a population as a cultural whole. The barriers to education and
prevention are very similar in all groups, but we concern ourselves with lan-

guage and culture differences, so we can fine-tune the message."

Other cultural considerations apply in the African-American community, according to Sherwood G. Dubose, special project administrator for Metro-Miami Action Plan:

> The fine-tuning in the black community is different. We don't
> have the communication system the Cuban community has.
> Who owns the medium of communication means a lot to the
> receiver. And, as a practical matter, whereas Dr. Laureano-
> Vega gets free public service announcement time on the
> Spanish stations, we have to pay on the black-programmed,
> white-owned stations. So we lose repetition, which is so
> important to a good education program.

Mr. Dubose says that another cultural factor to be reckoned with is a lack of trust in the system. "People in the black community perceive that the establishment here is still white, not Hispanic; that the white, moneyed group controls the community and tells the Hispanic public officials what to do."

In the Haitian community, "The concept of educating the family unit is the same as in the Hispanic community," according to Mireille Tribie, MD, deputy director of *La Liga Contra El SIDA*, a native Haitian who is married to Dr. Laureano-Vega. "But we have to work to get them to accept the fact that AIDS is what is affecting a family member. Many won't say the word and will deliberately misdiagnose what is wrong as, say, diarrhea."

Moreover, "Everything we do has to be by word-of-mouth," she says, "because of the low level of literacy. Here in Miami we are dealing with the 'boat people'—the farmers, mountain dwellers, and city people who had no education. We have to speak in Creole, since the majority of these Haitians do not speak French."

But Dr. Tribie has several things going for her. One, the Haitian community is geographically concentrated. Two, it relies on the woman to head the family in emergencies and illness. Three, Dr. Tribie has a lot of energy and a flair for communicating ideas:

> An educator and I go to beauty parlors in Little Haiti and ask
> permission to make a presentation. The owners like the idea.
> This is a relaxed atmosphere, a female hangout with no men

around. It is a second home for the women. We talk about
AIDS; about how it is not something just Haitians get; about
how women can get it as well as men; about how we must
protect our future children. They welcome it. And they
spread the word among their friends. This approach empow-
ers them with knowledge. It is like a conversational lecture.
We can get very explicit. The younger Haitian women are not
as narrow-minded about sex as the older ones. We talk about
exotic ways of keeping their partners from resenting the
condom.

Dr. Tribie has been reaching men through general presentations at
PTAs and neighborhood groups, but not in isolated, male-only groups.
"Haitian men don't go to the barber shop as often as women go to the beauty
parlor," she says. "But they do go to soccer games, and we are thinking of cap-
turing them with invitations to see the eliminations for the 1990 World Cup,
which we cannot get even on cable down here. A local club is negotiating with
us to get it in by satellite. We would make AIDS presentations at these sessions."

Matching Message and Audience

Mimi Tribie has her counterparts in Broward County, and they have adopted
the suburban version of her beauty parlor conversational lectures: "safer sex"
parties, where women meet in homes and talk. "We show them how to use
condoms," Jasmin Shirley Moore says. "We find out what their attitudes are
and those of their mates. And finally, we talk about how a woman can put her
foot down and refuse to have sex without protection."

She notes that in Broward County, "A trend is developing toward one
partner, monogamy, safer sex, and other prevention techniques. We should
consider that a breakthrough." As one sign of this, the Broward project is getting more requests from community groups for educational presentations and
has set up a program to prepare clergy to counsel their congregants.

Broward makes special informational efforts with the wealthy corporate community. Katie Kahrs Sanchez says:

I don't talk so much anymore about AIDS the disease when
talking to corporations and the straight community. I talk
about its economic impact. That gets their attention, they
start thinking, the fear and phobia start lessening, and they
can start understanding the predicament of people with AIDS.
They are prepared at this point to understand when I ask
them hypothetically, 'If I were going to take away your insurance, your house, and your car, would you tell me that you
had AIDS?'

Some professionals who deal with AIDS and other sexually transmitted
diseases approach sexuality in a clinical way, others are more pragmatic.
Workers in the Belle Glade project say that, in their community, "For many of
the males, to be sexually active is a very primary, basic thing, a form of suste-
nance as important as food and water. And that interferes with their ability to
keep themselves healthy."

In New York City, Ernest Drucker does not picture AIDS as a time
bomb, ticking away inside society. "It's more like a steady leak," he says. "Over
time, normal patterns of sexual contact will spread AIDS as it does every other
sexually transmitted disease."

Just at the time we need to consider human sexuality openly, he
believes, "American attitudes about human sexuality are going backward. It is
becoming more and more difficult to talk about sex." As a result, we are dis-
armed when it comes to dealing with something insidious like AIDS. "Sex is
rapidly becoming a more important method of transmission than needle use.
Needle-sharing is going to be aberrant; but sex is continuous. Drug injections
are the principal sexual vector for transmission to the non-addicts."

Michael McCord in Fort Lauderdale draws on the relatively successful
history of HIV education efforts among gay white men. "We deal with sexual
activity in the gay white male population, but there we are working for the most
part with educated people. In the minority communities, we often are not."

"Here and across the nation, this problem of sexual promiscuity is very
real," says one black physician. "I know that blacks are not supposed to talk
about it. But we must."

Education for Drug Users

Grady Hospital's Bob Parrish says, "I don't believe that we will ever create an education program here in Atlanta or anywhere else that drug addicts will find acceptable. Why? Because of the lifestyle that puts them there in the first place. Addicts are full professors of con artistry."

In Newark, Oswaldo Fierro holds the view that addicts are not afraid of AIDS, because "addicts are not afraid of death. They don't really care. Substance abuse is not an isolated fact in their lives, remember. Addicts share in a group. The sharing of blood is a part of the ceremony and social ritual of taking drugs together." Still, he believes that due to many factors, he is obtaining some results from efforts to change attitudes and behavior among drug addicts. "From the things that I hear, addicts are beginning to listen and share information about sexual practices. This is a tremendous change. But it is very slow, and you have to be very patient."

Bill Lafferty, MD, chief of epidemiology and surveillance for HIV/AIDS and infectious diseases in the Washington State Department of Health, acknowledges the extent of the feeling of helplessness that pervades AIDS services professionals when it comes to addicts. But he recalls that some people felt the same way about persuading gay men to change their behavior. "The AIDS model requires you to act without all the information and apply these techniques to the treatment of drug addicts," he says.

"The drug education problem may go back to that other lesson we learned from AIDS: you must treat the whole person, the mind as well asthe body," says Ernest Drucker.

Although between 75 and 80 percent of the Long Island Association for AIDS Care's case load has some kind of drug dependency, Jonathan Silin, PhD, LIAAC's former director of education, does not spend much time on drug use in his educational efforts. Instead, he focuses on changing behavior that is unsafe. "We tell people to learn from the gay community: how sexual practices can be changed; how to adapt to the situation; how to convince other people that safer sex is the norm. We tell them, 'The survival of your community depends on safer sex.'"

New York City is trying to address a drug problem so big it eclipses the AIDS epidemic. Drug use is the number one method of HIV transmission in the city. Among intravenous drug users, the New York City AIDS Task Force reported, the epidemic has been underreported. Officials are not thinking just about intravenous drug users, but also people who use crack. Crack is so addictive and so cheap that it is hastening the spread of HIV to women and teenagers, who offer sex in exchange for drugs or the money to buy them. Sex—not crack—is the method of transmission, but the drug is the impetus for sex with multiple partners.

Michael Baker sees a few faint rays of hope. City health department studies show that drug users are aware of the risk of HIV infection. Anecdotal information suggests that they are changing their behavior. But the change is uneven across groups.

Mr. Fierro says, "Now that drug users see people dying, their behavior is changing a little bit. Fourteen people have died around us in the past two years. That has a tremendous impact."

Education for Children

Educating children about AIDS is a controversial education and outreach task, because it involves teaching children about sex, something that many Americans believe should be done solely within the home.

At a New York City residential center for young runaways, an AHSP coalition member, a seroprevalence study found about 7 percent of the clientele is HIV-positive. "It's mostly sexually transmitted among these kids, but it's related to crack abuse," says a counselor there. Teaching safer sex is not the right response. The youngsters are knowledgeable, and they are frightened, but when they take drugs they are very likely to have sex. "We have to deal with their addiction. There is a horrible irony in the fact that the crack and AIDS epidemics hit young people simultaneously."

Across the river in Jersey City, Jack Cox thinks the ultimate solution is massive education for young people. "Look at those with high-risk behavior first. Start with children of addicts. In Newark, we have mothers, daughters, and granddaughters using drugs.

"We have to start in kindergarten and help kids learn how to deal with things that upset them emotionally. Unchanneled emotional outbursts very often trigger drug use."

In addition, he suggests:
- honest information about drugs and the progression of addiction
- special attention to the transition from eighth grade to high school ("a danger-

ous period—inevitably that was the pivotal year for the addicted kids I have dealt with")

- places where a parent can bring a child and have a drug-screening test done free, and
- a solid sports and physical education program.

Whether one's audience is drug users, gay white men, children, families, or the community at large, certain fundamentals apply, according to Dr. Silin of LIAAC. "First, education has to be repeated. People need time to think about these issues and come back to them again. Second, people open up to this issue only when they are personally affected, whether by AIDS in a family member, a neighbor, or a fellow worker. When that happens, they become receptive."

CLIENT ADVOCACY

Buren Batson has advocated actively on civil rights issues for both gay and straight people. But he firmly believes that issues of homosexual rights and the rights of the dispossessed are secondary to an AIDS health services project and that espousing them hinders fulfillment of its primary objective. When he took over as AID Atlanta's executive director, he wanted a clear board mandate "to make AID Atlanta a human services delivery agency that runs efficiently, no longer a political agency."

Still, he believes the agency should serve as an advocate for the client—regardless of gender or sexual preference—but not through political action. Some of the client advocacy needs cited by staff at the Belle Glade AIDS clinic, for example, are housing and support on legal issues, like guardianship. Another is confidentiality. "It's amazing how many of our own rules we break all the time," William Case, MBA, executive director of New York City's People With AIDS Coalition, says. "How often people's trust is compromised. Confidentiality is so easily broken that there is little faith that institutions will keep their word. If I went to a doctor to get an AZT prescription and had it filled at a local drug store, I believe that insurance companies all across the country could know about it immediately."

Gail Barouh of the Long Island Association for AIDS Care (LIAAC) describes her stand on this issue:

The best chance for survival for an AIDS organization is not to be seen as a gay organization. Our slogan is 'We Care for Everybody.' Yet, we must advocate for people who are discriminated against.

You can't turn your back on the gay community. If it weren't for the gay community, there wouldn't be an AIDS service program. Your volunteers are either going to be gays and lesbians or heterosexuals who are open to gays and lesbians. But, your board shouldn't be overwhelmingly anything. You have to represent the whole community. But, we adopted the policy of giving service to anyone who presented himself or herself for service.

Mr. Case, a financial marketer who left the New York Stock Exchange to become director of the People With AIDS Coalition, says that discrimination against people with AIDS "is one of the things that is going to make it harder and harder as we go on, because the epidemic is going to reach deeper into the ranks of the underprivileged. There will be less and less support for doing something about it and about them." Advocacy, then, is essential.

There are many different ways to advocate for the needs of a person with HIV or AIDS. Rather than a prescribed set of practices, advocacy is more a state of mind, in which providers are constantly serving as client advocates, just as they are constantly serving—consciously or unconsciously—as health educators.

Seattle's approach to advocacy is the most systematic in the 11 AHSP sites. A systems analyst studies problems that case managers have in obtaining services for their clients and identifies the root of the problem in regulations, laws, budgets, or agency practices. This information then becomes the basis for negotiation with the agency in question. If a change in law or regulation is needed, the responsibility transfers to the program's director, who may decide to seek a change in the law, calling in the Northwest AIDS Foundation legislative consultant in Olympia for assistance.

Ray Pople described how he and his 12 teams of AID Atlanta volunteers serve as advocates. The volunteer Practical Support Group works at Grady Hospital, as well as in clients' homes. One group works nights, one days.

According to Mr. Pople:

The care at Grady is wonderful now, but it took us three years
of teaching the hospital staff how to deal with our clients.
Initially they were resentful, even of giving us a gown for a
patient. Here we were giving our time, and we were getting
no support.

The augmenting of care we do now is more in providing emotional support and in helping an overworked staff
in a very busy hospital: feeding people, getting people up,
giving bed baths. We've forgiven them for having treated us
that way, and they've forgiven us for having yelled at them.

Another aspect of advocating for people with AIDS is recognizing how
isolated AIDS patients can become—how bereft of the support and help that
people generally take for granted—and stepping in to take action. Mr. Pople
said, "Three years ago people arrived on our doorstep with cardboard boxes
with all their effects in them—thrown out by family, landlords, or, in some
cases, lovers."

In Miami, the People With AIDS Coalition and The Body Positive, a
community center for people with AIDS, combine their role as advocates for
people with AIDS with the role of hosts for regular social activities, called
Positive Teas. "The people who are doing the best, healthwise, are the people
who are involved," says Jeffry Feinberg, vice president of the People With AIDS
Coalition of Dade County.

The same message comes from Michael McCord of Broward County.
"The People With AIDS Coalition was founded here a year ago to help people
survive longer. Relating to other people with AIDS helps with that. We give
one another mutual support and encouragement." Mr. McCord and his counterparts elsewhere put a great deal of emphasis on wellness programs, exercise,
diet, ways of reducing stress, and social events, which they find a good way of
drawing out people with AIDS.

According to a Seattle AIDS caseworker, clients have said that all their
lives they never had any friends, and now they have so many.

Chapter 8
PROBLEMS AND STRATEGIES FOR PROJECT FINANCING

Programs that provide HIV-related care and services need sufficient financial resources for ongoing operations, as well as start-up expenses. Without adequate funding, programs don't thrive, services are threatened, and people in need of HIV care suffer in various ways. In the 1990s, funding mechanisms for HIV-related programs and the people they serve are precarious and ever-changing, especially as implementation of the Ryan White law proceeds. Providing a comprehensive account of strategies to secure funding for AIDS care is beyond the scope of this book. This chapter highlights some of the early experiences of AHSP projects as they confronted the challenges of financial survival.

The Robert Wood Johnson Foundation made it clear from the outset that its funding of the AIDS Health Services Program was for project development and not ongoing support. The Foundation urged grantees to develop alternative sources of long-term funding for the comprehensive array of services needed, but the projects have found this difficult. In general, hospital care is covered by public or private insurance (or hospitals provide the care without reimbursement), ambulatory services are covered less well, and community-based services—like housing or social services—are usually not covered at all. State Medicaid eligibility and reimbursement rules—or low rates of physician payment—hinder access to services. Nevertheless, AHSP grantees have made progress in generating financial support through both service reimbursement arrangements and fund-raising.

Gary W. Swisher, director of public information and AIDS education for Oak Lawn Community Services in Dallas, has learned a lesson in both psychology and long-term funding: "Value your services; don't give them away.

Don't let people with AIDS come to you with the attitude that you owe them something. Don't set yourself up to go broke."

Typically, grant-funded projects assign future funding plans a lower priority than immediate program needs; in the AIDS field, where immediate needs are often crises, attention to the short-term is particularly understandable.

Yet, strategic planning is vital for acquiring resources and developing funding mechanisms that enable AHSP projects to move towards financial self-sufficiency, and is equally important as determining specific client service needs. Without adequate attention to long-term survival, consortia are ill-prepared to expand their services or adapt to changing community needs.

The problems of financially sustaining service programs for people with AIDS are made extraordinarily difficult because of the extreme poverty of the clientele. "I don't think people realize the great indigency involved in the AIDS population," Betsy Pegelow of Dade County says:

> They should see the difficulties caregivers run into in the homes. We are supposed to be doing high-tech work, and we find ourselves having to set up our own food bank and hold a drive to get donations of bleach. Basic physical sustenance is not there in so many cases—I mean people don't have clothes to wear, pots to heat food in, something to heat a frozen meal in. No bleach.

A Palm Beach CAP case manager says, "This epidemic has opened my eyes to some social and economic realities in the United States. Until you go into your first crack house to evaluate a patient, you don't understand what you have read and heard about poverty."

Among the Broward Hospice case load, no greater than 2 percent still have insurance to pay for their care. Carole Shields, administrator of the AIDS program for Hospice, Inc., in Miami, explains:

> We have got to find a way to spread the financial risk around and not let the insurance companies off the hook. My staff routinely has to spend a whole day putting the heat on an insurance company that has cancelled a patient's medical insurance. Then we will have to pay the premiums for his insurance out of one of our related organizations. Even

though hospice services would continue regardless, we have to work to protect the patient's insurance coverage, since a future acute care need might require that payer.

SERVICE REIMBURSEMENT

"AIDS is a hot topic now," Mary Boland of Newark's Children's Hospital says, "but when it no longer is, we will have to go back to the traditional funding system, which doesn't cover the kinds of non-traditional things we do in this program."

An important element of that system is Medicaid. For example, the hospital cannot bill Medicaid for outpatient nursing services or social worker services provided by the case manager unless a child is in a special Medicaid waiver program. States determine whether to cover such services, and most don't. Fulfilling the typical reimbursement requirement that a physician be present when such services are rendered would be both logistically difficult and extremely costly.

Dallas physician Philip O'Bryan Montgomery is clear about the effects of Medicaid's limited coverage for outpatient care: "Parkland Hospital has to admit people when they don't need to be hospitalized. They could be taken care of in an apartment house. If we don't do something about Medicaid, we will cause Parkland to endure considerable debt."

Two AHSP projects—Seattle and New Jersey—have made headway in tying down significant funding from government sources. In both cases, the projects set their sights on the governmental level next up the line: Seattle took aim on the State of Washington; New Jersey on federal health and welfare programs.

Seattle worked with state officials to obtain funding for sheltered housing set up by the project and, with other Washington cities, convinced the legislature to establish an AIDS network that makes modest monies available for care and treatment. Additionally, the Northwest AIDS Foundation, the city's partner in the AHSP project, has been outstandingly successful in raising private money for its education and service activities.

Seattle

Money is used sparingly and creatively in Seattle to hold together the beginnings of a permanent, comprehensive system of treatment and services to people with AIDS and an extensive program of community and individual education and counseling aimed at preventing the spread of HIV infection.

In addition to the AHSP project funded by The Robert Wood Johnson Foundation, Seattle taps at least eight other major sources of program funding, not including funds contributed by local and state service and religious entities:

- A four-year grant from the federal Centers for Disease Control (CDC) supports a wide range of activities: HIV antibody testing and counseling, outpatient primary care, AIDS education to high-risk groups, including school curriculum development, and a long-term research study of high-risk group members. CDC, through the state Department of Social and Health Services, also supports an active AIDS surveillance system.
- The federal Health Resources and Services Administration awarded the health department a three-year, $1.2 million grant to supplement the AHSP project begun with funds from The Robert Wood Johnson Foundation.
- The National Institute on Drug Abuse supports the project's AIDS prevention efforts among intravenous drug users and their sexual partners.
- The federal Medicare (disability) and federal-state Medicaid programs pay for health services under established rules governing eligibility and benefits.
- The state Medicaid plan has been amended not only to include case management as a reimbursable service but also to permit local funds to be used to match federal funds. Customarily, because Medicaid is a state-federal program, state funds make up this match.
- Seattle-King County receives a share of money appropriated by the state legislature to prevent and control AIDS and to establish a regional AIDS Service Network.
- The City of Seattle and King County together contributed nearly $470,000 to the AIDS Prevention Project in 1989, slightly lower than their 1988 contributions.
- The Robert Wood Johnson Foundation separately supports a demonstration project to design and test AIDS education interventions among people engaging in recreational drug and alcohol

abuse and high-risk sexual practices.

- *In fiscal year 1988-1989, the Northwest AIDS Foundation raised $867,000 in individual contributions and an additional $133,000 in corporate contributions. In addition, the value of the more than 70,000 volunteer hours contributed to all the organizations in the AIDS network was estimated at more than $420,000 annually.*

New Jersey was the first state to obtain a federal waiver that permits the state to use Medicaid funds to buy home care and community-based services for people with AIDS. This allows individuals with diagnosed AIDS-related illnesses to receive extensive care in the community as an alternative to nursing home or hospital inpatient care.

Although the Medicaid waiver applies to only a subset of HIV-infected individuals whose poor health requires an institutional level of care, for those who have met the eligibility criteria—some 1,400 by the fall of 1990—a wide range of community-based services (including payments of $125 per month per client for case management services) is covered: case management, private-duty nursing, medical day care, personal care assistant services, certain narcotic and drug abuse treatments at home, hospice care, and intensive supervision for children who reside in special foster homes.

Other states might want to pursue such waivers, despite their strict financial eligibility criteria, but should do so, advises New Jersey AHSP Director Steven Young, "only after getting a good handle on how many people need what kinds of services and the extent to which they have (or potentially have) Medicaid coverage."

Both these efforts are of the scope that the Foundation had in mind when discussing with grantees the need to secure future funding.

Mr. Swisher believes, "The state, the county, and the city are going to have to pitch in financially. They have to do more than ride herd on outside money. Corporations are going to have to start making contributions of money and people. Just about any health service agency is going to have to accommodate AIDS in its program," and will face the consequent need to secure financing for these services.

New York State, likewise, has developed a wide variety of funding and service initiatives. A prominent example is legislation that gives greater Medicaid reimbursement—as much as one and one-half times the usual daily rate—to hospitals designated as regional referral centers for people with AIDS.

Hospitals located in high AIDS-incidence areas can apply to become designated as AIDS centers. Both inpatient and outpatient medical services for people with AIDS, as well as case management services, must be provided through these centers. Presumably, designation helps hospitals achieve some economies of scale in providing this range of services, by increasing the number of AIDS patients seeking treatment. Thus far, primarily the voluntary hospitals have pursued designation; some hospitals, unable to comply with designation regulations (stringent staffing requirements, for example), do not seek designation despite their location in high AIDS-incidence areas.

As one of these regional referral centers, the Nassau County Medical Center must offer "a comprehensive array of services, and in turn, we get $788 per day instead of $550," David Jaffe says. The additional referrals "build our census, which reinforces our designation and helps us do our job as a member of the AIDS consortium better."

Differential reimbursement provides an incentive for hospitals to stay involved in AIDS care, in the face of a number of incentives to minimize such activities. Many hospitals fear the stigma of the "AIDS hospital" label, if their inpatient case loads of people with AIDS increase disproportionately to other inpatient admissions. Furthermore, people with AIDS put an enormous strain on hospitals when they seek hospitalization simply because they have nowhere else to turn, because adequate community-based services do not exist.

A 1987 survey of hospital losses associated with caring for people with AIDS, funded by The Robert Wood Johnson Foundation, demonstrates that all hospitals—public and private—lose money on AIDS care. Yet these losses hit public hospitals much harder. A combination of serving patients who need higher-cost care and lower revenues for public hospitals—because they also tend to serve more Medicaid and uninsured patients—means public hospitals in the survey lost $218 for every day of AIDS care provided, more than twice the daily losses of private hospitals. The larger AIDS case loads that public hospitals serve simply compound this shortfall, as does their greater case load of pediatric patients with AIDS.

For Carole Shields of Hospice, Inc., of Broward and Dade Counties, pediatric AIDS illustrates the disease's crushing financial potential:

> Getting these kids out of Jackson Memorial Hospital and into
> a home is critical in terms of managing costs. We had an
> infant 19 months old who had been in Jackson for all but a

couple of months of his life. Imagine the cost! His mother is a drug addict, but his father is stable, so with a little help, he could manage. Our intervention, which made it possible for the father to work and also care for the child, cost us $6,000. It would have cost Jackson $60,000 a year to keep him. In such cases, the value of comprehensive community-based services and family-centered case management is clear.

Regional differences in hospital losses are pronounced. In regions where Medicaid programs are more generous—like the Northeast and West—private hospitals treat more AIDS patients than they do in other regions, and their daily losses even exceed those of public hospitals. Where Medicaid programs are parsimonious, notably the South, public hospitals lose the most per day ($386). Still, for public hospitals in Northeast states, which treat the largest number of intravenous drug users, even more generous Medicaid programs cannot offset the major overall losses attributable to AIDS care. Like their southern counterparts, each public hospital in the Northeast lost some $600,000 on AIDS care in 1987.

Study Director Dennis P. Andrulis, PhD, (president of the National Public Health and Hospital Institute in Washington, D.C.), also underscores the ominous concentration of AIDS hospital services: less than 5 percent of hospitals provide more than 50 percent of AIDS care. These and other hospitals serving disproportionate numbers of poor and uninsured people with AIDS will be thrust inevitably into economic crisis.

One solution to these difficult circumstances may be for hospitals to adopt the community-based consortium approach. Nassau County Medical Center provides a successful model. By participating actively in the community-based consortium, Nassau County Medical Center can help assure that the full range of out-of-hospital services is in place and running smoothly, in order to prevent inappropriate hospital utilization.

AHSP projects that can demonstrate lower costs than conventional care may have a leg up in negotiating with potential funders. One of the goals of the AHSP was to show that providing a comprehensive array of outpatient and support services would provide an alternative to long-term hospitalization that would be not only more desirable for people with AIDS, but also less costly. Data on this latter issue so far are sparse, but there is anecdotal evidence that hospital lengths of stay have declined for AIDS patients in at least some AHSP project cities:

- Grady Hospital in Atlanta has reduced average lengths of stay for AIDS patients from 13 to 10 days, a trend attributed by Dr. Bill Elsea to more outpatient services for people with AIDS.
- In Seattle, Swedish Hospital Medical Center reports that the outpatient clinics that are part of the AHSP kept hospital days in the first year down to an average of 7.5 per patient. "It's good," says Ann Benson, RN, MBA, an infection control practitioner at the hospital. "But we would like to do better—we're limited by community resources."
- These figures compare favorably with national survey data indicating that in 1987 AIDS patients in public hospitals like Grady had average lengths of stay of 17.7 days and that the average number of hospital days per year for AIDS patients in private hospitals like Swedish is 26.

Not all the 11 communities have fared as well. In those cases where only small cost savings have been achieved, the single greatest barrier to progress was the lack of outpatient services, especially housing and long-term care.

Local AIDS projects can look beyond conventional health funding sources for both money and consortium members. For example, Glades Acts in Belle Glade, Florida, receives money from the county Department of Housing and Community Development, which in turn gets funding, in part, from the U.S. Department of Housing and Urban Development (HUD). As much as a quarter of this local agency's work is AIDS-related.

Bill Cooper, reporter for the Palm Beach *Post,* believes the county's Comprehensive AIDS Program (CAP) stands a good chance of getting money from both state and municipal government once it has established its reputation for handling its money soundly. "It takes more than good intentions to make people want to give you money," he says. "It takes financial sophistication and accountability."

Shauna Dunn, CAP's director, agrees and also is determined to mine better the sources of money already available. "The county could help us more. We could increase what we bill for nursing services and get a home health care agency license." At the time of her interview, she was considering taking the steps necessary to enable CAP services to be reimbursed by both Medicare and Medicaid.

FUND-RAISING STRATEGIES

As with reimbursements, having a variety of fund-raising sources and approaches can strengthen a project's flexibility and long-term prospects. Some AHSP projects have learned that having a foundation or government grant lends the credibility necessary to raise other funds successfully. Ideally, a project finds a balance between general contributions and the kinds of funding that bring strings with them.

Some community projects engage professional development planners to help their boards with fund-raising. For example, the Long Island Association for AIDS Care eased into fund-raising by persuading a major Long Island corporation to underwrite the salary of a fund-raiser, who prepared a three-year development plan that so far has been a success.

In most AHSP communities, fund-raising has been haphazard, but not unproductive. For example, CAP received almost $60,000 in unsolicited funds in one six-month period. However, during other time periods, both planned and unplanned solicitations have been much less fruitful. Shauna Dunn foresees more federal monies and expanded support from businesses and individuals. "If you have good relations and make good presentations, you get new people interested in the program, and you can raise money," she says.

Specialized publications that suggest funding opportunities for AIDS-related organizations can serve as a starting place for projects to develop their own fund-raising plans. For example, the New York AIDS Consortium supported development of a resource directory, *Guide To Funding For HIV/AIDS Projects*, prepared by Welfare Research, Inc., which identifies potential corporate, foundation, government, and civic support for New York City-based AIDS service providers.

Although Broward County's Center One did not put together its first formal fund-raising plan until the spring of 1989, it has been successful raising money from the community. Katie Kahrs Sanchez says, "Getting the 'wives of' involved is a good idea." Wives of prominent citizens are good at organizing and attending luncheons and other benefits. Such activities, she suggests, do more than just raise money:

> You get good public relations, and this increases the awareness level. The wives educate the community and the business leaders. Now that we have AIDS babies, they are—

unfortunately—an especially powerful subject for both fund-raising and public information. Gay people working in the design field have influenced their wealthy clients to give money, and that helps, too.

Mary Boland of Newark's Children's Hospital says, "Care and services money is the hardest money to get. People will give you all the money you want for education or research. But we need to get money down to where the patients are. It's not glamorous. It's never-ending. There's no product, nothing for funders to put their names on."

Rolando Rodriguez, executive director of the Catholic Health and Rehabilitation Foundation of Miami, also has run into problems trying to raise funds for AIDS treatment and services. "The combination of Spanish machismo and Southern fundamentalism is potent," he says, even among socially promi-nent people who normally are big givers. He reports in 1990, "a noticeable change in attitude. It's becoming much more okay to give and participate in AIDS causes—especially ours since it's associated with the Church." The women still lead the way, he says. "The men have a fear of being labeled as gay."

Competition for scarce charitable dollars can be fierce. For example, Mary O'Donnell, RN, MHM, associate director of Hospice Care of Broward County, says fund-raising efforts that draw money out of Broward County for Dade County programs pose a very real problem. "We need that money here. Some of this money is going to the University of Miami for research. I think the drug companies and others that typically fund research should be tapped first. I recognize that many Broward residents benefit from the research, but we are in urgent need of direct care dollars."

By contrast, Mr. Rodriguez has no problem when film-star Elizabeth Taylor and the American Foundation for AIDS Research raise money in Miami. "Their fund-raising here doesn't hurt us. In fact, it helps, by making giving to AIDS causes respectable."

IN-KIND CONTRIBUTIONS

Cure AIDS Now in Dade County hates to spend money. Almost all the provi-sions it supplies to people with AIDS are donated by a generous community, according to Director of Operations Marlene Arribas. Even the trucks and vans and refrigerators and shelving that constitute the delivery system itself are donated. So, too, is much of the labor that goes into boxing, sorting, driving, and telephoning. A lot of that comes from the agency's clientele, people with AIDS.

"Some clients want to work, to be busy," Ms. Arribas says. "It makes them feel better."

Volunteer Bob Grummons runs a food pantry for people with AIDS in West Palm Beach. "I've learned a lot, and every day something new," he says. "One thing is never to discount the love and support of the gay community. The food and money they give makes the pantry possible. Only 10 percent of my clients are gay, yet 95 percent of the operating funds come from the gay community."

He has found the rest of the community forthcoming, as well. Winn-Dixie, a supermarket chain, provided shelving for the pantry. Couples make contributions to mark their wedding anniversaries. Individuals give donations in memory of departed loved ones or as birthday presents for friends.

SIGNS OF PROGRESS

Finding the funds for client services has challenged the creativity of the AHSP projects. A number of innovative strategies have evolved that may be applicable in other communities. Federal regulations allow states to include case management as an optional service in their Medicaid programs, though many states still do not. When Washington officials wanted to add case management, they faced the problem that no state matching funds were available for this new service. As Alberta Larsen explains, "With federal, state, and local cooperation, we were able to take a creative approach. We now use local instead of state funds to match the federal money for case managers' services."

Working within religious and political constraints in a state with chronically underfunded public health and social welfare programs, Dallas's AIDS Task Force recommended that the city have a lay board to help coordinate funding requests on public health matters. They suggested that this board coordinate grant requests to foundations and to city, county, state, and federal agencies, in order to avoid overlapping requests and streamline processes. That has been accomplished. Says task force Chairman Dr. Montgomery, "Funders need and want the assurance that local people are not competing with each other for money. You have to get your act together." And, the imprimatur of the board helps their application.

The Washington State Risk Pool, like the Dallas public health board, is not just for people with AIDS. Newly formed, it is built on a straightforward idea: A person at risk of any disease and who has been rejected by an insurance company pays $60 a month for coverage by the pool. The risk pool program is thought to be ideal for HIV-positive people who are still able to work. Without significant premium subsidies from the state, lower-income people with catastrophic illnesses have been unable to take advantage of state risk pools, even where they exist. This financing option is still too new to have a track record of acceptability or performance for people with AIDS, but worth watching.

Health planners in Washington state are at work on another new program that would do something—at least temporarily—about the health care plight of the indigent, which most severely affects public hospitals. The kernel of the project is a proposal that other hospitals in the state contribute money or services to public hospitals, in order to help them cover the costs of providing indigent health care. Washington's largest public hospital, Seattle's Harborview, would be the main beneficiary. Without such help, health care professionals in Seattle concur, the hospital will not remain financially afloat.

On the federal level, the passage of the Ryan White Comprehensive AIDS Resources Emergency (CARE) Act of 1990 serves as the nation's first comprehensive AIDS care law. Signed into law in August 1990, the CARE Act offers some relief for several of the communities with AHSP projects, as well as others. The intent of this legislation is twofold: to make federal funds available to metropolitan areas hardest hit by the HIV epidemic by helping to meet immediate needs; and to offer support to states for developing early intervention and other services for people with HIV living in less affected areas where resources are limited.

The CARE Act has four discrete components. Title I establishes an HIV Emergency Relief Grant Program for metropolitan areas disproportionately affected by the HIV epidemic (defined as having more than 2,000 AIDS cases reported to the Centers for Disease Control or an incidence of 25 AIDS cases per 100,000 residents). In fiscal year 1991, 16 metropolitan areas were eligible to receive this assistance; seven of the nine communities served by AHSP projects met these eligibility requirements. Title II makes HIV Care Grants available to states for the work of HIV care consortia, home- and community-based care, health insurance coverage, and provision of treatment. Title III provides assistance to states to expand early intervention and HIV prevention services. Title IV encourages the development of pediatric demonstration projects, establishes federal health services research priorities, and outlines various guidelines for programs to train emergency response employees (fire, police, emergency medical personnel) in communities.

Of the $350.5 million appropriated through the CARE Act, only $144 million represents new federal dollars. Ranging from $100,000 to $13.8 million per state, most of the funds that states will receive through this legislation are from existing federal programs that have been merged into the CARE Act (such as the AIDS drug assistance program and programs to encourage home- and community-based care). Nevertheless, this legislation is a significant development that is consistent with the basic tenets of the AHSP, by supporting a comprehensive approach to HIV-related care and services and encouraging community-based organizations and local, state, and federal government entities to work together in coordinating services and meeting financial needs related to HIV care.

Chapter 9
THE MEDIA:
OBSERVER OR PLAYER?

Coverage by the news and information media affects an AIDS services project's ability to attract and keep patients and volunteers; it plays some role in furthering a project's community education goals; it can either help establish or detract from a project's credibility and leadership in the community, and thereby affects its ability to forge institutional alliances and raise funds. In the long run, media coverage may warm or cool a project's prospects for survival.

AIDS, like many complex problems that beset society, is difficult for the media to cover consistently and well. Although dramatic medical and scientific breakthroughs are popular among news editors, they are rare. Routine news about the delivery of AIDS services is intrinsically less interesting, particularly so now that the initial novelty of the disease has passed. Many editors apparently deem this kind of AIDS coverage a low priority.

According to data recently compiled by the federal Centers for Disease Control (CDC), the number of stories about AIDS and HIV found in 100 selected publications declined significantly in the late 1980s. Although the number of people diagnosed with AIDS continues to increase substantially each year, print media stories dropped roughly 50 percent in 1988-1989, when compared with a peak of 11,852 stories recorded by CDC in a similar survey in 1987.

"Media attention to AIDS is down lately," Dr. Manuel Laureano-Vega confirmed for Miami in May 1989. "This produces the perception on the street, 'Oh well, AIDS must be going away, because I don't hear about it so much any more.' That is not the case!"

Despite the recent decline in the number of AIDS news stories, a 1989 study conducted by The Wirthlin Group (an American survey and polling firm) and Hill and Knowlton, Inc., (an international public relations and public affairs company) suggests the potential for a resurgence in media attention. Their study reveals that "an overwhelming majority of health and science reporters nationwide cite AIDS as the dominant healthcare story of the '80s and believe that it will continue to dominate health news in the '90s."

These findings were verified in news reporters' and editors' responses to a 1989 opinion survey conducted by Healthcare Communication Systems, Inc., for The Robert Wood Johnson Foundation. Health care reporters, editors of professional health care journals, and reporters and editors at news services, newspaper syndicates, and national news periodicals identified AIDS as the leading health care topic. Syndicate editors and newspaper reporters ranked AIDS public policy and AIDS medical treatment first or second in a list of 27 varied health care topics. Only telecasters ranked AIDS policy significantly lower (10th). Organizations dedicated to meeting the needs of people with AIDS may find a receptive audience among reporters and editors, if they are approached correctly.

AHSP project staff in Broward County see the press as an ally. This may account for—or result from—the good coverage the project and Center One have received. Veronica Ostrandes, Center One's former volunteer resource coordinator, says, "The more media you get, the more volunteers you get. There has been a great deal of positive publicity about Center One and about AIDS, and it has brought us a terrific number of straight women volunteers." One broadcast netted 20 calls the next day from people interested in volunteering.

"To get in the straight press you need your tokens: babies, anonymous professionals, women—usually not showing their faces and with their voices distorted," she says. "Anything but a gay white male."

When members of the local press are not well acquainted with the local gay community, they may take the easy route—find a few visible spokespeople from advocacy agencies and consistently turn to them for their views. If these individuals are hostile to a particular project, the results may be damaging. In such situations, projects that already have established good relationships with reporters find them more likely to give the project spokesperson an adequate opportunity to respond. The result is a better, more balanced story.

"Always remember," advises AHSP media consultant Andrew I. Burness, president of Burness Communications, "a crisis is not the time to develop a media strategy."

Instead, The Robert Wood Johnson Foundation has tried to help prepare its AHSP project directors for interactions with the media in several ways, aimed in part at avoiding crises and, in part, at coping with them if they come.

- Media training for project directors, including a short course on crisis communications.
- On-site technical assistance for project directors. Depending on their particular needs and preferences, a wide range of services was made available, including assistance in the development of a media plan, advice on what to look for in hiring a communications staff person, ways to strengthen relationships among staff of consortium-members' own public relations offices and the AHSP project, project-specific media training for staff, and strategic planning for working with the local media.
- Publication of *AIDSline,* a quarterly newsletter circulated to AHSP grantees and a large number of other individuals and organizations working in the AIDS field, providing current information and news story ideas.
- A step-by-step guide on how to work with the media.
- Problem-solving sessions at annual meetings of grantees, providing advice on questions involving the media.

AHSP communications consultant Mr. Burness offers the following specific tips to guide the media relations activities of project directors in community-based AIDS organizations:

- Look for free help where you can get it. Make contact with a major public relations firm in your area, or ask who to contact at the local chapters of the Public Relations Society of America and the International Association of Business Communicators. Also, look for student volunteers from local colleges or retired executives. Since your time is limited, look elsewhere for low-cost expertise.
- Develop accurate press lists, so that when you want to inform the local press about an event or a news item, you will know where to reach them. This can best be done by working collaboratively with the public relations office of other consortium institutions (including hospitals, health departments, and universities).
- Identify the five to 10 key journalists in the community who cover AIDS, and keep them apprised of your activities. As a general rule, try to meet with one reporter each week. If you do, you will meet with each of them every two to three months. These regular backgrounders will cement relationships, diffuse the mystery of the reporter-newsmaker relationship, simplify matters when your organization chooses to seek coverage proactively, and provide ideas that reporters may turn into feature stories.

- Make secondary use of press clippings and television segments. For example, when a favorable article appears in the newspaper, neatly duplicate it, and send it to prospective funders, legislators, board members, and others who would be impressed. Never let a flattering article or broadcast piece sit on a shelf. Seek the broadest exposure possible for your good news.
- When meeting with a reporter, understand that anything you say may be quoted. There is no such thing as "off the record," whatever the reporter tells you. Consequently, be careful, but don't be so uptight that the spirit of your message is lost. The best interviews are conversations, not stilted, jargon-laden one-liners.
- Never say "no comment" to a reporter's question. You have three choices: "I know the answer, and here it is"; "I don't know the answer"; or "I know the answer, but I'm not in a position to tell you, and here's why." A fourth option is to try to avoid conversation on a topic that you would rather not address.
- To supplement publicity about your project, generate media attention by writing occasional opinion pieces for your local newspaper or arrange to comment on your local television or radio station. You are not solely dependent on the whims of editors; if they don't find your message interesting, then go straight to the public through the editorial pages and broadcast commentaries.
- Always remember that "news" is just that—it is new. Your organization's acquiring a new treasurer or your speaking at a local church is not news. A new survey on the extent of the epidemic in your community or a celebration of The Names Project in your state capital is news. Your credibility with the press is directly related to your understanding of what makes news. As a rule, if it is truly interesting, it is news. If it's ho-hum, more of the same, it's not news.
- When you have "news"—that is, a truly groundbreaking story—share it with all reporters on your list. A press conference may not be necessary if someone is prepared to stand by the phone and answer questions (work out good answers to ticklish questions in advance).
- Be very selective when you seek a correction in the newspaper or in the broadcast media. Virtually every story will have at least a minor inaccuracy. And any objective profile of your organization will not be entirely flattering. (You can turn that situation around if you let the reporter know you agree with the critique and say how your organization intends to rectify the prob-

lem. A positive follow-up story may ensue.) Save your letters-to-the-editor or calls to the reporter or producer for egregious errors that give an entirely false impression of your project.

- Be on the lookout for any opportunities to generate local news attention by tagging onto a national news event. For example, when CDC releases its nationwide report on the incidence of AIDS, local projects could highlight statistics from their area.

- Likewise, if a project has a relationship with a better-known entity, a direct connection with this entity should be clearly stated. For example, "State officials in Governor X's cabinet will be receiving testimony today from (local project director) about the unmet needs of people with AIDS."

- Remember that you are speaking for your organization. Consequently, the organization must have a united position. This does not mean that you need to call a board meeting before responding to a press inquiry, but that your expressed views are indeed "collective" and not merely your own personal opinions. All staff who deal with the press should stick to "the party line," and, ideally, the staff who do speak to the press should do so only with the approval of the project director.

- Media relations activities should be tightly controlled. A project director should know about any media contact before it happens. Designating one central spokesperson promotes continuity and efficiency. When an organization issues a statement or is approached for an interview, an additional spokesperson should be included only when that person truly has something valuable to add and can offer increased credibility with regard to a specific issue. For example, a lawyer can speak with authority about legal matters confronting an organization or a physician can offer expertise on relevant medical problems.

Some AHSP project directors have taken the initiative by calling key reporters, introducing themselves by identifying their organization as a major provider of AIDS services in the city, and simply saying, "I'd like to meet with you to talk about what's happening with the AIDS epidemic in our city." Usually reporters agree.

"Establishing relationships that are straightforward, natural and conversational is key; hype doesn't work, and projecting a purely businesslike tone puts reporters off," says Mr. Burness. He adds that each project spokesperson should be prepared with a one- or two-sentence phrase in concise layman's terms that answers the request, "Tell me about your organization and what it does."

In Dallas, the AHSP project spokesperson has established mutually beneficial relationships with local media professionals. Special efforts have been made to inform fully editorial columnists and editorial boards of the two Dallas daily newspapers about AIDS, leading to editorials on critical topics. In part as a reaction to these editorials, county government created a planning commission on AIDS.

In Seattle, the media listened to both the mayor and representatives of the gay community who paid calls upon them. Not only did they cover the story of the AHSP project, they joined other employers in adopting personnel policies that benefit their employees with AIDS.

Developing and implementing an effective media relations plan requires careful consideration and some expertise. Given the time constraints and lack of media relations experience of many AIDS project directors, one approach is to organize a board communications committee. This advisory committee could include at least three people: a public relations person from an AIDS consortium institution, a public relations person working for a firm in the community, and a journalist. Meeting quarterly, the committee could assist staff (or even a volunteer) designated to serve a communications role by providing advice on proposed publications and media interactions and by generating ideas for media opportunities.

Good coverage of an AIDS health services project requires a broad view, because of the variety of issues these projects confront every day: the need for political leadership, improved insurance coverage, revamped public assistance and housing programs, private-sector participation, and public awareness.

A national organization deeply concerned about public understanding of AIDS is the National Commission on Acquired Immune Deficiency Syndrome. Thomas D. Brandt, the Commission's director of communications, makes a number of positive suggestions regarding increasing public understanding of the epidemic:

- The epidemic is moving into the black, Hispanic, and other minority communities, and proportionately more women and children are becoming infected. This new dynamic opens new journalistic areas. While overall AIDS coverage in the press is diminishing, projects that deal with these newly affected communities have the "fresh angle" that is critical to competitive journalists. Of course, stories about minorities also may help a program reach these tradition-ally difficult-to-reach populations.
- Project officers often overlook the single best resource they may have in com-

municating with the news media—the Person Living With AIDS. The media initiative that includes PLWAs who are available to the press and representative of the issues will often have a better response from the media. "Human interest" is the key. That being said, using PLWAs requires absolute sensitivity to issues of confidentiality and good advance planning. Work out the "ground rules" with PLWAs in advance on issues like identification or describing their circumstances, insure that journalists are aware of and agree to these preconditions, then tightly monitor the event to insure compliance.

- An effective way to enhance media coverage of your initiatives is to have select opinion leaders outside your organization briefed in advance so they will be willing and able to make favorable public comments. Before announcing a new program or releasing a report, that means giving "embargoed" copies to important people in your area like the mayor, congressman, school or health officials, and others.

- A primary media relations tool can be an organization's Fact Sheet. It can include basic information on who you serve, your objectives, your staff, members of your board, budget, sources of financial support, and how you fit into the fabric of social service in your community. If crisply written, the Fact Sheet will be welcomed by journalists for their background files. It will improve the accuracy of their stories and will help keep you in mind as a source of information on HIV. Easily updated, it is a ready reference to answer general information requests and to make available when your group meets publicly or when your officials make public appearances or give speeches.

The first step for AHSP projects in achieving working relationships with the news and information media has been to recognize their potential importance to the project and the need to work with them effectively. In any case, the nature of AIDS and its impact on people and society makes working quietly, out of the limelight, almost impossible.

Steven Sternberg is one of seven full-time science writers for the Atlanta *Constitution,* and he covers the AIDS beat for the paper. He finds the news stories he covers about AIDS are not just medical stories or scientific ones, but stories about the community's social and financial infrastructure, as well. "The people in DeKalb and Fulton Counties are supporting Grady Hospital with their taxes. So AIDS is costing them. They don't realize that, and they don't realize the changes in the demography of the disease."

Critically important in its own right, AIDS also has brought to light problems in the health care system that affect a great many Americans not infected with HIV. Says Mervyn Silverman, director of the AHSP:

> It has become a truism to say that AIDS is a metaphor for the problems in the health care system and society in general. The only things new about AIDS are the virus and the fact it primarily affects people in the prime of their lives. We can only hope that the lessons learned in fighting AIDS can be used to transform our nation's health and social service systems in ways that benefit us all.

People Mentioned in the Text

In general, the titles and affiliations used in the text and listed here are those from the time interviews were conducted. Sometimes a different title is provided because it better explains a person's relationship to the project.

Andersen, Heather A.
RN, MN
Training and Curriculum Specialist, AIDS Education and Training Center
    Program, University of Washington
Former Clinical Director, Hospice of Seattle
Seattle, WA

Andrulis, Dennis P.
PhD, MPH
President, National Public Health & Hospital Institute
Washington, DC

Arribas, Marlene
Director of Operations, Cure AIDS Now, Inc.
Miami, FL

Baker, Michael
MD
Acting Assistant Commissioner, Division of AIDS Program Services,
New York City Department of Health
New York, NY

Barczykowski, Sister Anthony
DC (Daughters of Charity)
Chief Executive Officer, Associated Catholic Charities of New Orleans
New Orleans, LA

Barouh, Gail
MA
Executive Director and Chief Executive Officer,
Long Island Association for AIDS Care, Inc.
Huntington Station, NY

Batson, Buren
Consultant
Former Director, Atlanta AIDS Health Services Program project, and
    Former Executive Director, AID Atlanta, Inc.
Atlanta, GA

Benson, Ann
RN, MBA
Infection Control Practitioner, Swedish Hospital Medical Center
Seattle, WA

Bianchi, Barry
Board Chairman, Northwest AIDS Foundation
Seattle, WA

Boland, Mary G.
RN, MSN
Director, AIDS Program, Children's Hospital of New Jersey
Newark, NJ

Brandt, Thomas D.
Director of Communications,
National Commission on Acquired Immune Deficiency Syndrome
Washington, DC

Brown, Marjorie T.
MD
Chief, Personal Medical Services, Dade County Public Health Department
Miami, FL

Buckingham, Warren W., III
Project Director, Dallas AIDS Health Services Program project, and
    Executive Director, AIDS ARMS Network, Inc.
Former Associate Director, Community Council of Greater Dallas
Dallas, TX

Burness, Andrew I.
President, Burness Communications
Bethesda, MD

Byers, Tom
Former Aide to Seattle Mayor Charles Royer
Seattle, WA

Bykonen, Margo
RN
AIDS Outpatient Coordinator, Swedish Hospital Medical Center
Seattle, WA

Byrnes, Claudia
MSW
Associate Executive Director, Community Council of Greater Dallas
Dallas, TX

Calkins, Al
Co-Founder, Lesbian/Gay Political Coalition
Dallas, TX

Campagna, Pat
Coordinator, Housing and Social Services,
Long Island Association for AIDS Care, Inc.
Huntington Station, NY

Carmichael, Lynn
Chief, Family Practice Service, Jackson Memorial Hospital, and
    Professor and Chair, Department of Family Medicine and Community Health,
University of Miami School of Medicine
Miami, FL

Carr, Jane C.
RN
Director, Office of Infectious Disease, Georgia Department of Human Resources
Atlanta, GA

Case, William
MBA
Executive Director, People With AIDS Coalition
New York, NY

Collier, Ann
MD
Medical Director, AIDS Clinic, Harborview Medical Center, and
    Assistant Professor of Medicine, University of Washington
Seattle, WA

Cooper, Bill
Reporter, Palm Beach *Post*
West Palm Beach, FL

Cox, Jack
MA
Director of AIDS Services, Spectrum Health Care
Jersey City, NJ

Dodds, Sally
Director, AIDS Health Crisis Network
Miami, FL

Dornan, Douglas
MS
Consultant, Home Health Care
Former Executive Director, AIDS Resource Center
New York, NY

Drucker, Ernest
PhD
Director, Division of Community Health, Montefiore Medical Center
New York, NY

Dubose, Sherwood G.
Special Project Administrator II, Metro-Miami Action Plan
Former Director of Training, Metro-Dade Transit
Miami, FL

Dunn, Shauna
RN, MS
Director, Palm Beach AIDS Health Services Program project, and
    Executive Director, Comprehensive AIDS Program of Palm Beach County, Inc.
West Palm Beach, FL

Elsea, Bill
MD, MPH
Commissioner of Health, Fulton County Health Department, and
    Professor of Preventive Medicine and Community Health,
Emory University Medical School
Atlanta, GA

Feinberg, Jeffry
Vice President, People With AIDS Coalition of Dade County
Miami, FL

Fierro, Oswaldo
Executive Director, C.U.R.A.
Newark, NJ

Fullwood, P. Catlin
Executive Director, People of Color Against AIDS Network
Seattle, WA

Grummons, Bob
Director, Palm Beach County Food Pantry
West Palm Beach, FL

Gumbart, Conrad H.
MD
Chairman, Metropolitan AIDS Advisory Committee, and
    Associate Professor of Medicine, Louisiana State University
New Orleans, LA

Guthrie, Kevin
Director, Volunteer Services
Long Island Association for AIDS Care, Inc.
Huntington Station, NY

Haigney, John
Director, Client Services
Long Island Association for AIDS Care, Inc.
Huntington Station, NY

Hannon, Philip M.
President, WLAE (a Catholic broadcasting station)
Former Head of the Archdiocese of New Orleans
New Orleans, LA

Iacino, Dick
MA
Deputy Director, Center for Adult Development and Aging,
University of Miami
Miami, FL

Jaffe, David E.
MPA
Director, Nassau County AIDS Health Services Program project, and
    Chief Operating Officer, Nassau County Medical Center
East Meadow, NY

Joseph, Steven C.
MD
Dean, School of Public Health, University of Minnesota
Former Health Commissioner, City of New York, and
    Chair, New York City AIDS Task Force (1989)
Minneapolis, MN

Kaetz, Susan
MPH
Research Consultant, School of Public Health, University of Washington
Former Director, AIDS Education and Training Center, University of
    Washington
Seattle, WA

Kator, Mark
Executive Director, Coler Memorial Hospital
Roosevelt Island, NY

Kelly, Sister Mary Louise
RN, PHN, MSA
Former Executive Director, Nursing Sisters Home Visiting Service, Inc.
Brooklyn, Nassau, & Suffolk Counties, NY

Kruzich, Andy
Director, New York City AIDS Health Services Program project, and
    Director of Program Development, New York AIDS Consortium
New York, NY
Former Project Coordinator, Seattle-King County AIDS Health Services
    Program project
Seattle, WA

Lafferty, Bill
MD
Chief, Office of Epidemiology and Surveillance,
HIV/AIDS and Infectious Diseases, Washington State Department of Health
Seattle, WA

Landrieu, Mitch
State Assemblyman, District 90
New Orleans, LA

Larsen, Alberta
RN, MN
Nurse Consultant/Advisor,
Washington State Department of Social and Health Services
Olympia, WA

Laureano-Vega, Manuel
MD, MS
Founder and Executive Director, *La Liga Contra El SIDA*
Former Health Educator, South Florida AIDS Network
Miami, FL

Lebedynec, Maria
Case Manager, St. Michael's Hospital
Newark, NJ

Lee, Philip R.
MD
Director, Institute for Health Policy Studies,
University of California, San Francisco, School of Medicine
San Francisco, CA

Levine, Steven
MBA
Assistant Hospital Administrator/Grant Manager,
    Nassau County Medical Center
East Meadow, NY

Lomax, Rebecca
MPH, PhD
Administrator, AIDS Health Services Program project,
Associated Catholic Charities of New Orleans
New Orleans, LA

Long, Bill
Co-Chairperson, People With AIDS Coalition
West Palm Beach, FL

Love, Juliette
Former Director, Center One
Fort Lauderdale, FL

Loyd, Barbara King
Director, Miami AIDS Health Services Program project, and
    Administrator, South Florida AIDS Network
Miami, FL

Martelli, Becky
Special Projects Coordinator,
Washington State Department of Social and Health Services
Seattle, WA

Martin, Jim
Member, Georgia House of Representatives, District 26
Atlanta, GA

Mason, Abbott
Administrative Services Coordinator,
Comprehensive AIDS Program of Palm Beach County, Inc.
West Palm Beach, FL

McCord, Michael
President, People With AIDS Coalition
Broward County, FL

McInturff, Patricia
MPA
Director, Seattle AIDS Health Services Program project, and
    Director, Regional Division, Seattle-King County Department of Public Health
Seattle, WA

Michaels, Glenna
Health Policy Consultant
Former Director, New York City AIDS Task Force
New York, NY

Montgomery, P. O'B., Jr.
MD
Professor of Pathology, University of Texas, Southwestern Medical Center, and
    Chair, AIDS Task Force
Dallas, TX

Moore, Jasmin Shirley
MSPH
AIDS Patient Care Director, Broward County Public Health Department
Fort Lauderdale, FL

Moos, Bob
Editorial Writer, Dallas Morning *News*
Dallas, TX

Mor, Vincent
PhD
Director, Center for Gerontology and Health Care Research, Brown University
Providence, RI

Morrison, Clifford
MS, MN, RN, FAAN
Deputy Director, AIDS Health Services Program,
Institute for Health Policy Studies, University of California
San Francisco, CA

O'Donnell, Mary
RN, MHM
Associate Director, Hospice Care of Broward County, Inc.
Former Director, Bereavement and Education,
Hospice Care of Broward County, Inc.
Fort Lauderdale, FL

Osborn, June E.
MD
Chair, National Commission on AIDS, and
    Chair, National Advisory Committee for the AIDS Health Services Program
Washington, DC

Ostrandes, Veronica
Former Volunteer Resource Coordinator, Center One
Broward County, FL

Paris, Nancy M.
Vice President, Saint Joseph's Mercy Care Corporation, and
    Chair, Board of Directors, AID Atlanta, Inc.
Former Vice President, Visiting Nurse Foundation
Atlanta, GA

Parrish, Bob
Associate Director, Grady Memorial Hospital
Atlanta, GA

Pate, Larry D.
MPA, NHA
Administrator, Padua Community Services (part of Catholic Charities)
Former Director, New Orleans AIDS Health Services Program project
New Orleans, LA

Pegelow, Betsy
RN, MSN
Assistant Director, Medicare Alzheimer's Project
Former Director of Special Projects, Visiting Nurse Association of Dade County
Miami, FL

Philbin, Pat
RN
AIDS Care Coordinator, Group Health Cooperative of Puget Sound
Seattle, WA

Plummer, Phil
Administrator, Jackson Infant & Toddler Shelter Home
Former Administrator, South Florida AIDS Network
Miami, FL

Pople, Ray
Former Volunteer Coordinator, AID Atlanta, Inc.
Atlanta, GA

Rodriguez, Rolando D.
MS
Executive Director, Catholic Health and Rehabilitation Foundation
Miami, FL

Royer, Charles
Director, Institute of Politics, John F. Kennedy School of Government,
Harvard University
Former Mayor of Seattle
Cambridge, MA

Sanchez, Katie Kahrs
Program Development Coordinator, Somerset Treatment Services
Former Case Manager, Center One
Fort Lauderdale, FL

Shields, Carole
Administrator, AIDS Program Hospice, Inc.
Miami, FL

Sievert, Alan J.
MD, MPH
Director, Division of Physical Health, DeKalb County Board of Health
Atlanta, GA

Silin, Jonathan
PhD
Former Director of Education, Long Island Association for AIDS Care, Inc.
Huntington Station, NY

Silverman, Mervyn F.
MD, MPH
Director, AIDS Health Services Program, and
    President, American Foundation for AIDS Research
San Francisco, CA

Smith, Don
PhD
Chief Psychologist, Georgia Mental Health Institute
Atlanta, GA

South, Rev. Kenneth T.
MDiv
Executive Director, AIDS National Interfaith Network
Former Director, AID Atlanta, Inc.
Atlanta, GA

Sternberg, Steven
Reporter, The Atlanta *Constitution*
Atlanta, GA

Stoddard, Thomas B.
JD
Executive Director, Lambda Legal Defense and Education Fund, and
    Adjunct Associate Professor of Law, New York University
New York, NY

Swisher, Gary W.
Director of Health Services, Oak Lawn Community Services
Dallas, TX

Thurman, Sandra L.
Director, Atlanta AIDS Health Services Program project, and
    Executive Director, AID Atlanta, Inc.
Atlanta, GA

Tribie, Mireille
MD
Deputy Director, *La Liga Contra El SIDA*
Former Director, Miami Hemophiliac Treatment Center
Miami, FL

Ward, Bob
MSW
Executive Director, North Miami Community Mental Health Center
North Miami, FL

Wiewora, Ron
MD, MPH
Medical Director, AIDS Clinics, Palm Beach County Public Health Unit
West Palm Beach, FL

Wilber, Joseph A.
MD
Medical Consultant, Office of Infectious Disease, Division of Public Health,
Georgia Department of Human Resources
Atlanta, GA

Young, Steven R.
MSPH
Director, New Jersey AIDS Health Services Program project, and
    Director, Care and Treatment Unit, Division of AIDS Prevention & Control,
New Jersey State Department of Health
Trenton, NJ

For Notes

For Notes